# LONG TRAILS
# OF THE
# SOUTHEAST

# LONG TRAILS OF THE SOUTHEAST

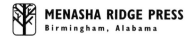

**MENASHA RIDGE PRESS**
Birmingham, Alabama

*This book is for Lisa Ann Daniel, who takes hikes*

Library of Congress Cataloging-in-Publication Data

Molloy, Johnny, 1961–
     Long Trails of the Southeast / by Johnny Molloy.
         p. cm.
     ISBN 0-89732-530-3
     1. Hiking—Southern States—Guidebooks. 2. Southern States—
Guidebooks. I. Title.

GV199.42.S66 M65 2002

                                                                    2002024446

Cover design by Bud Zehmer
Text design by Reider Publishing Services
Cover photos by Johnny Molloy
All other photos by Johnny Molloy

Menasha Ridge Press
P.O. Box 43673
Birmingham, Alabama 35243
www.menasharidge.com

# CONTENTS

# ACKNOWLEDGMENTS

Thanks to John Cox, Ellie Connolly, Aaron Marable, Chris Phillips, and Bryan Delay for hiking long trails with me. Y'all made writing this book a lot less like work. Thanks to my brother, Pat, for letting me stay with him down in Sylva Rena, Mississippi, and taking me grappling before hiking the Black Creek Trail. Thanks to all the rangers of our Southern national forests for answering lots of questions about the long trails in their districts. Thanks to Pat and Terry Gibbs of Black Creek Canoe Rental down in Brooklyn, Mississippi, for their help and generosity, and to the folks on the bulletin board at alabamatrail.org for all the helpful advice on the Pinhoti Trail. Thanks to Lisa Daniel for helping keep me organized from afar. Thanks to my old friend Cisco Meyer for running shuttle and camping out with me on the Foothills Trail in South Carolina. And thanks to Bud Zehmer and the folks at Menasha Ridge Press for their input. Thanks to the folks at Eureka! for providing me with watertight tents and Camp Trails for supplying quality backpacks that went every foot of every trail.

Each spring, thousands of backpackers head for Georgia to attempt a thru-hike of the Appalachian Trail. Many thousands more simply satisfy themselves with weekend or week-long jaunts along sections of the trail. And while the AT is a beautiful place, hiking along this trail without encountering many groups of people is becoming increasingly difficult to appreciate. In a word, the AT experience has changed; it has become more about community in the outdoors than a remote and solitary adventure. This is not bad—it's probably more in line with Benton Mac-Kaye's original intention for the trail—but it can still be rather disconcerting for a hiker expecting a solitary outing to discover 20 other cars at the trailhead.

Living in the shadow of the Smoky Mountains for over two decades, I have never been far from the Appalachian Trail. I have also been fortunate that my vocation as an outdoor writer has allowed me to spend time on the AT and other places. While I have yet to thru-hike the entire trail, I have backpacked the AT through the Smoky Mountains numerous times, staying at all of its shelters. I've also followed segments passing though Mount Rogers National Recreation Area and Shenandoah National Park. I have observed the increasing popularity of the trail first hand. Some time ago, I began wondering if there weren't other quality long trails in the Southeast to be hiked, trails that weren't so busy. The seeds of this book were sown.

The other motivation behind this book was the realization that many people do not have the time or desire to hike the entire 2,000-plus miles of the AT, yet they still want to get away on a long trail and get a taste of what hiking long distance is like. In response to the above, I researched and explored the trails included in this guidebook.

My first "research" occurred way back in 1988, during a multi-day backpack on the Pinhoti Trail of Alabama. I found the steep wooded slopes of the Talladega National Forest just as beautiful as anything I had found in the Smokies. Over the years, I discovered other long trails, including the Florida Trail and Benton MacKaye Trail, often while researching other books. I even found one of the hikes in this book, the Black Creek Trail, while on a canoe trip in Mississippi. Eventually the book came into focus and became a reality. It was a challenging and ultimately rewarding experience. Along the way I met trail maintainers and other avid long trail hikers who were seeking the same experience this book offers: a chance to hike and backpack long trails just as rewarding yet lesser traveled than the Appalachian Trail.

Just like life in the big city, life on the trail wasn't always great. I swatted more than a few mosquitoes on the Black Creek Trail, got drenched in a deluge of thunderstorms on the Benton MacKaye Trail, and hiked in the sun during a winter heat wave down Florida way. But these experiences were spices in the entrée. I also saw dogwoods in bloom on the Wild Azalea Trail, the fall colors from atop Stone Mountain on the Bartram Trail, and the froth of Whitewater Falls on the Foothills Trail. With this guidebook in hand, I hope that you will get out on the long trails of the Southeast and make some memories of your own.

# Map Legend

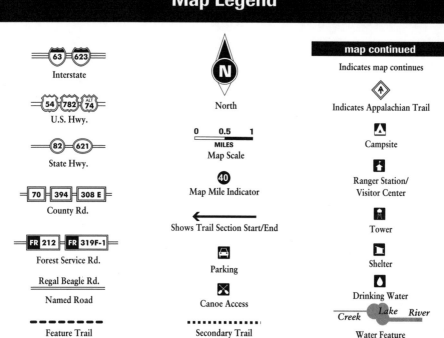

**Interstate** 63 623

**U.S. Hwy.** 54 782 74 ALT

**State Hwy.** 82 621

**County Rd.** 70 394 308 E

**Forest Service Rd.** FR 212 FR 319F-1

Regal Beagle Rd.
**Named Road**

**Feature Trail**

North

0 0.5 1
MILES
**Map Scale**

40
**Map Mile Indicator**

**Shows Trail Section Start/End**

**Parking**

**Canoe Access**

**Secondary Trail**

**map continued**
Indicates map continues

Indicates Appalachian Trail

**Campsite**

**Ranger Station/
Visitor Center**

**Tower**

**Shelter**

**Drinking Water**

Creek  Lake  River
**Water Feature**

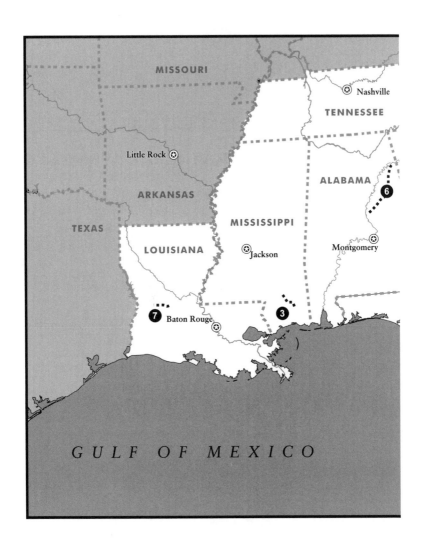

GULF OF MEXICO

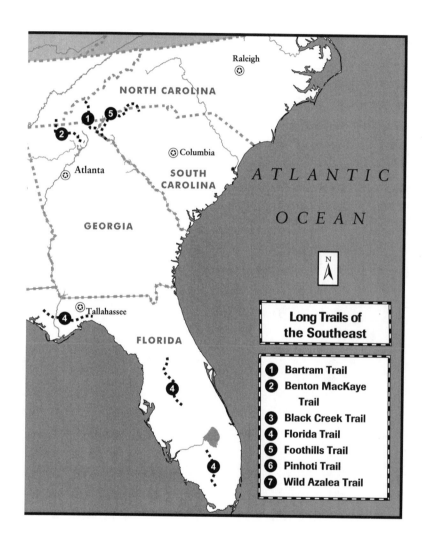

Raleigh

NORTH CAROLINA

Columbia

SOUTH CAROLINA

Atlanta

GEORGIA

ATLANTIC

OCEAN

N

Tallahassee

FLORIDA

**Long Trails of the Southeast**

1 Bartram Trail
2 Benton MacKaye Trail
3 Black Creek Trail
4 Florida Trail
5 Foothills Trail
6 Pinhoti Trail
7 Wild Azalea Trail

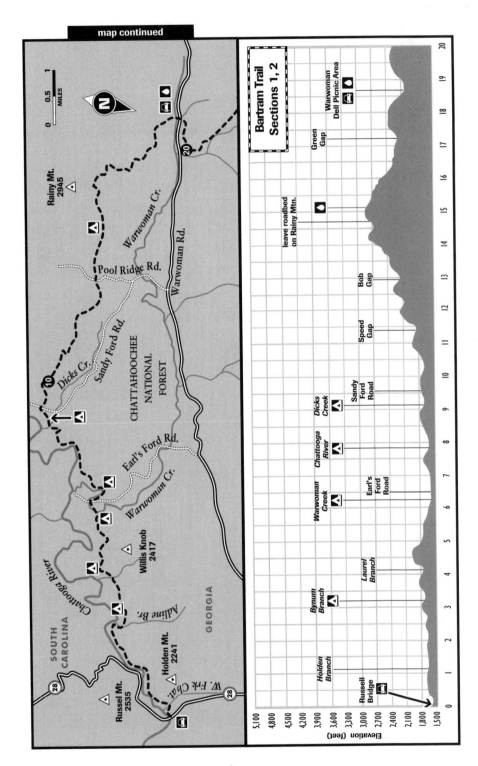

Bartram Trail
Sections 1, 2

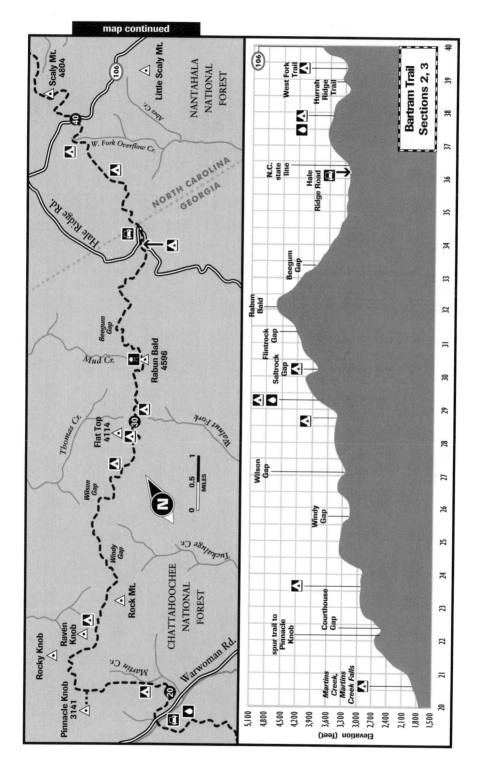

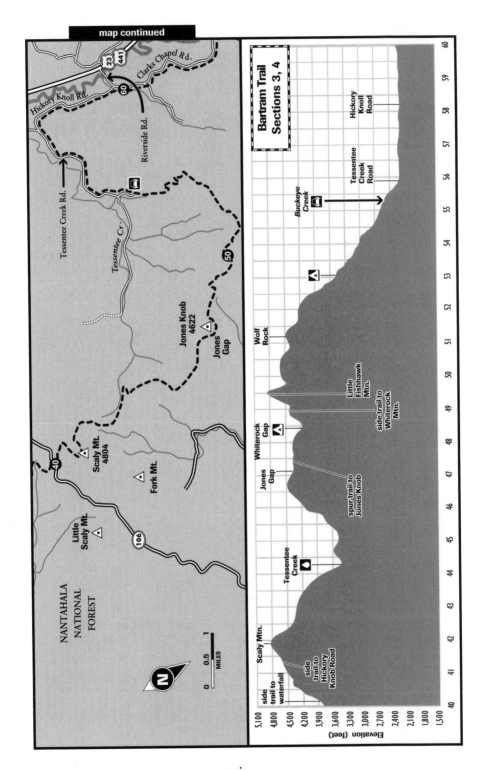

Clarks Chapel Rd.

Hickory Knoll Rd.

Riverside Rd.

Tessentee Creek Rd.

Tessentee Cr.

Jones Knob
4622

Jones
Gap

Scaly Mt.
4804

Fork Mt.

Little
Scaly Mt.

NANTAHALA
NATIONAL
FOREST

N

0    0.5    1
MILES

## Bartram Trail
## Sections 3, 4

Hickory
Knoll
Road

Tessentee
Creek
Road

Buckeye
Creek

Wolf
Rock

Little
Fishhawk
Mtn.

side trail to
Whiterock
Mtn.

Whiterock
Gap

Jones
Gap

spur trail to
Jones Knob

Tessentee
Creek

Scaly Mtn.

side
trail to
Hickory
Knob Road

side
trail to
waterfall

Elevation (feet)

5,100
4,800
4,500
4,200
3,900
3,600
3,300
3,000
2,700
2,400
2,100
1,800
1,500

40   41   42   43   44   45   46   47   48   49   50   51   52   53   54   55   56   57   58   59   60

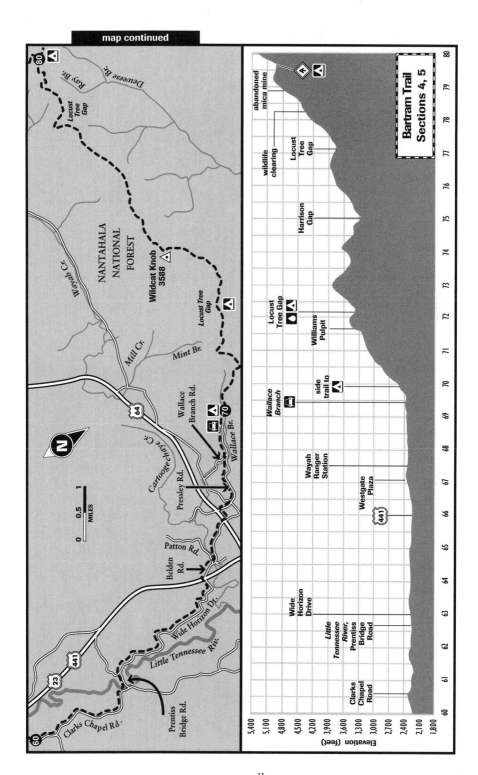

Bartram Trail
Sections 4, 5

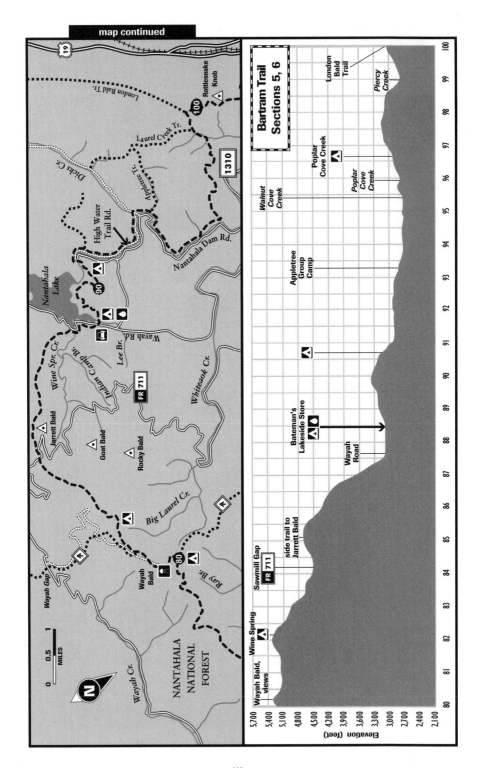

map continued

xviii

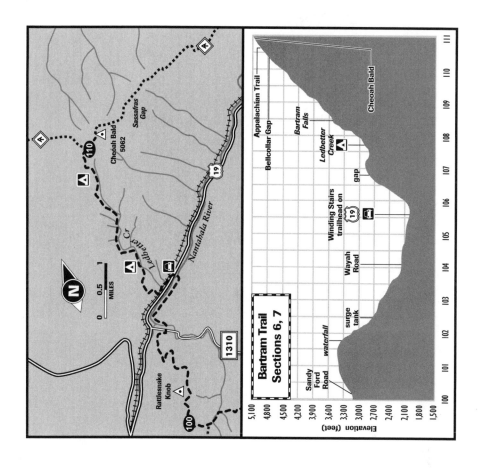

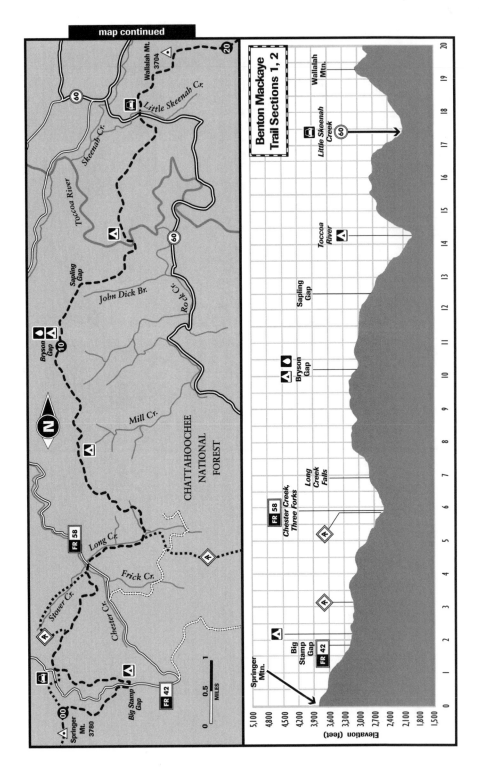

Benton MacKaye
Trail Sections 1, 2

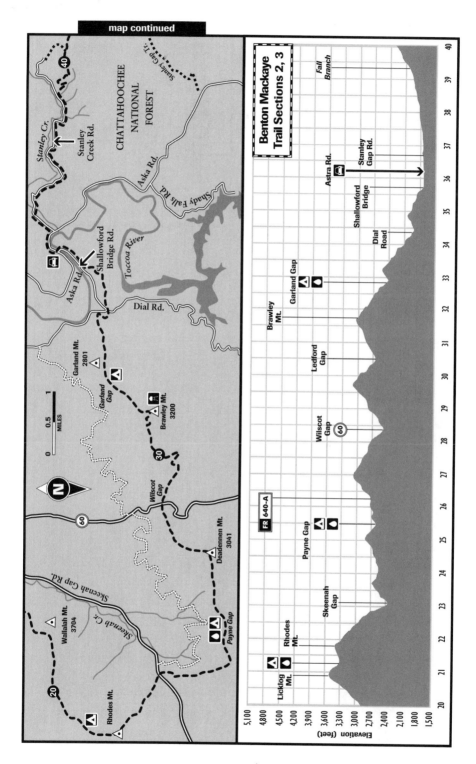

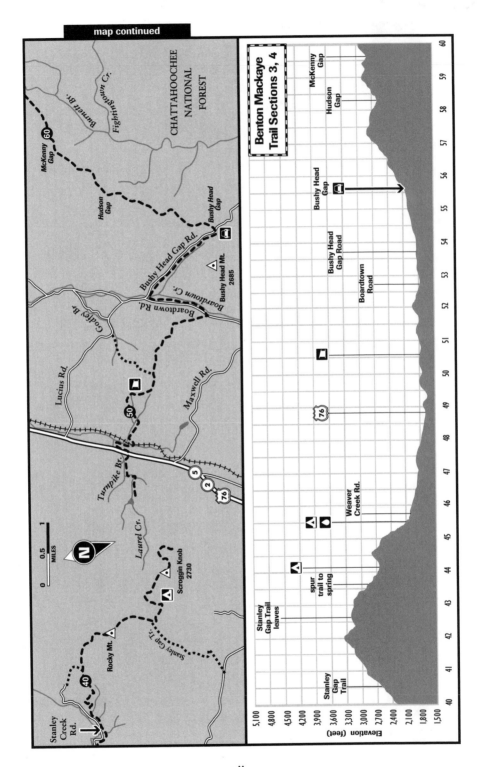

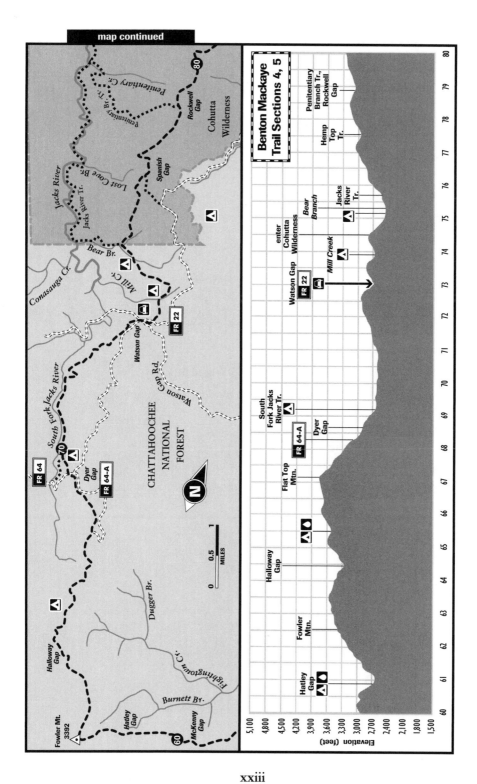

Benton Mackaye
Trail Sections 4, 5

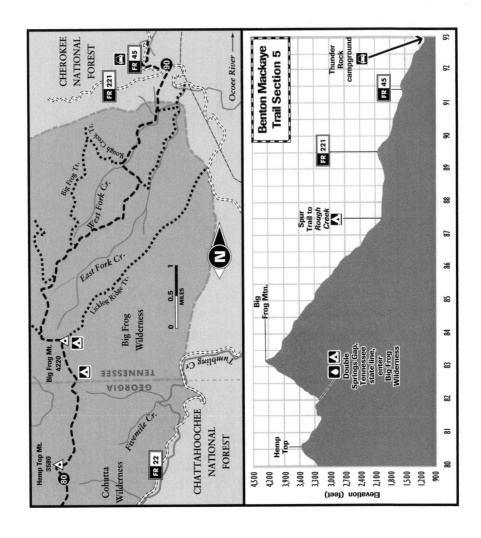

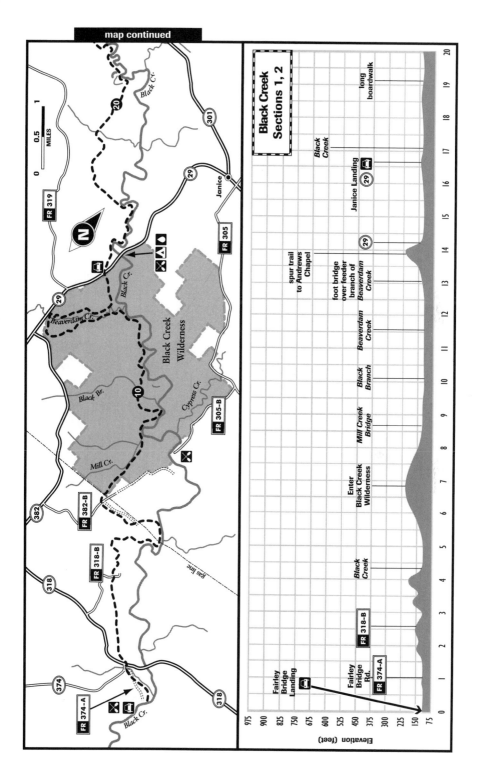

xxv

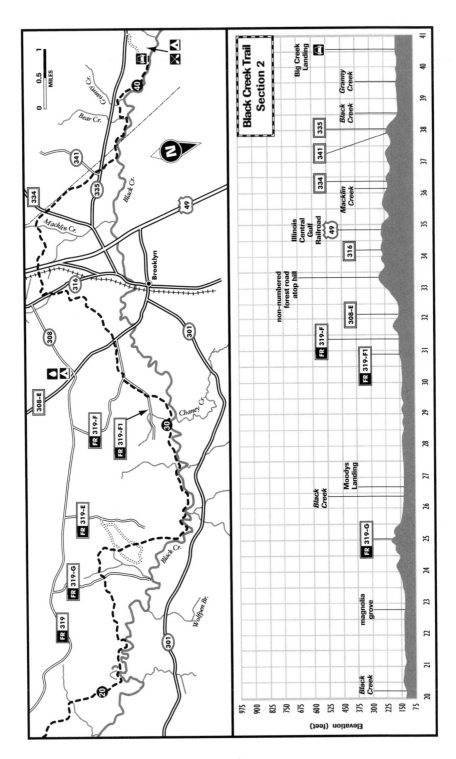

Black Creek Trail
Section 2

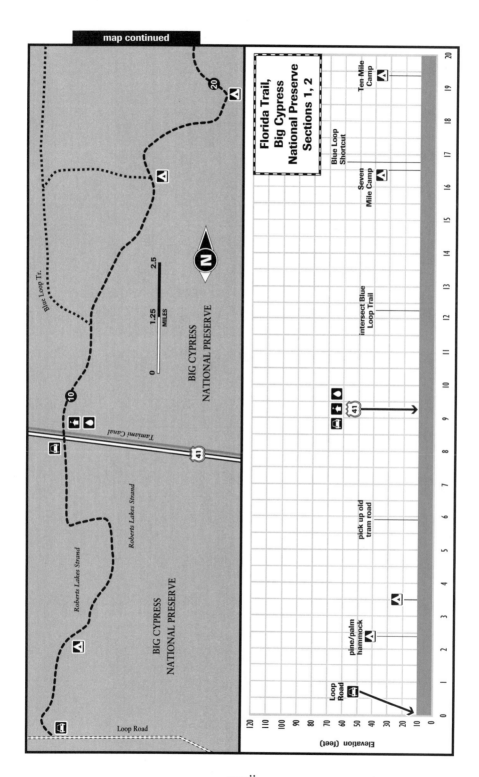

Florida Trail,
Big Cypress
National Preserve
Sections 1, 2

BIG CYPRESS
NATIONAL PRESERVE

BIG CYPRESS
NATIONAL PRESERVE

Blue Loop Tr.

Roberts Lakes Strand

Roberts Lakes Strand

Tamiami Canal

Loop Road

N

MILES
0    1.25    2.5

Ten Mile Camp

Blue Loop Shortcut

Seven Mile Camp

intersect Blue Loop Trail

pick up old tram road

pine/palm hammock

Loop Road

Elevation (feet)

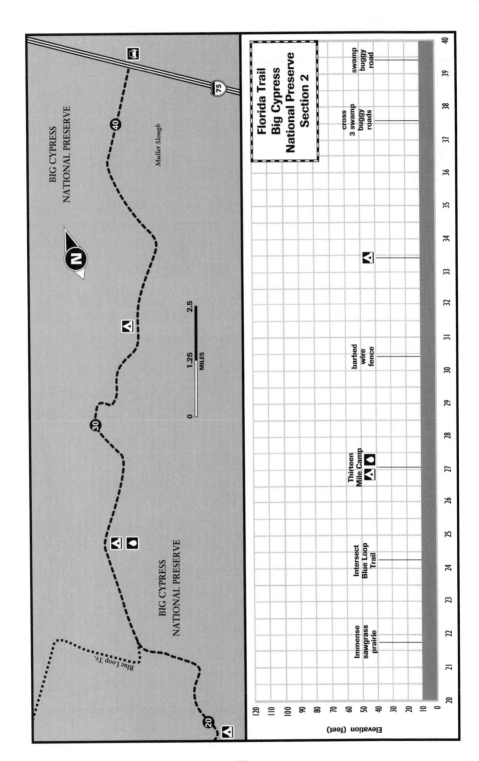

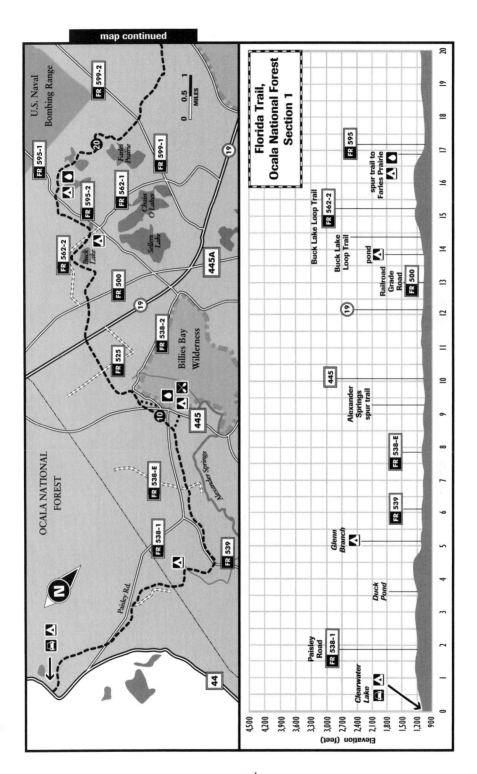

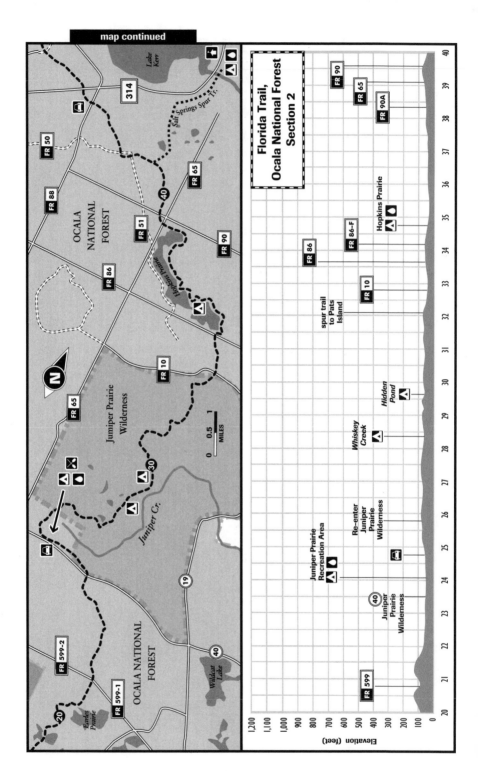

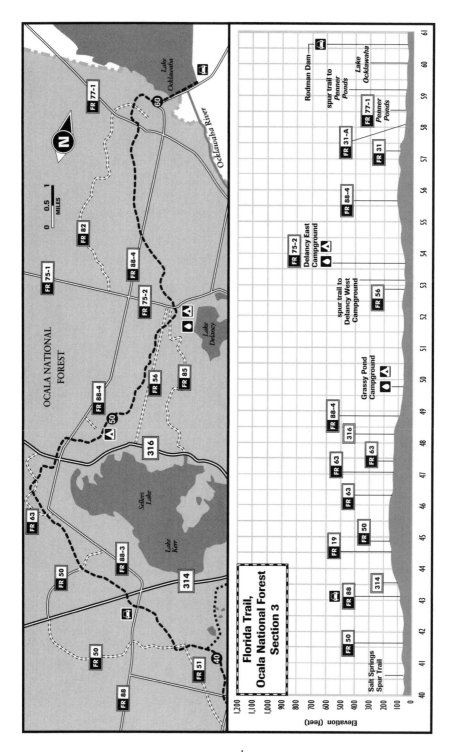

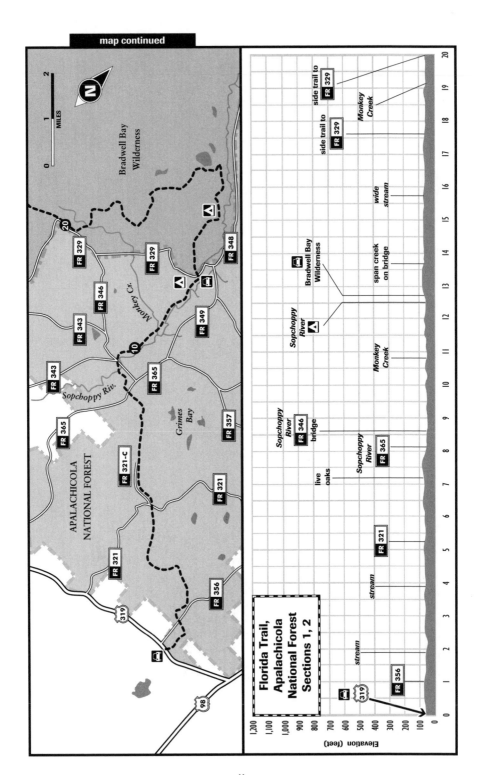

Florida Trail,
Apalachicola
National Forest
Sections 1, 2

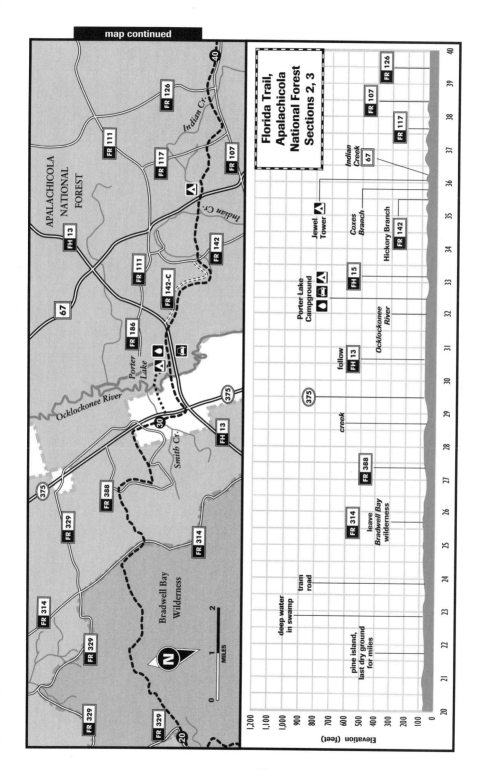

Florida Trail,
Apalachicola
National Forest
Sections 2, 3

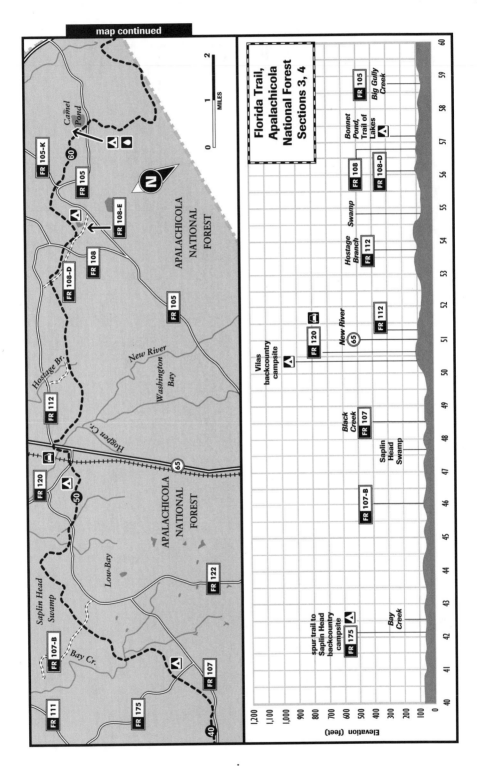

Florida Trail, Apalachicola National Forest Sections 3, 4

APALACHICOLA NATIONAL FOREST

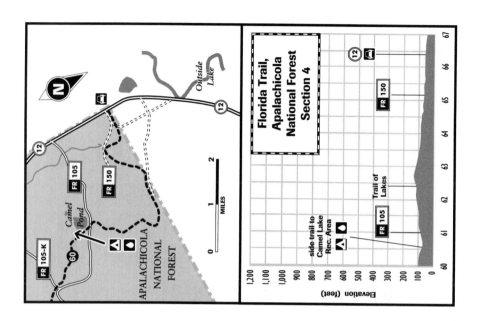

Florida Trail,
Apalachicola
National Forest
Section 4

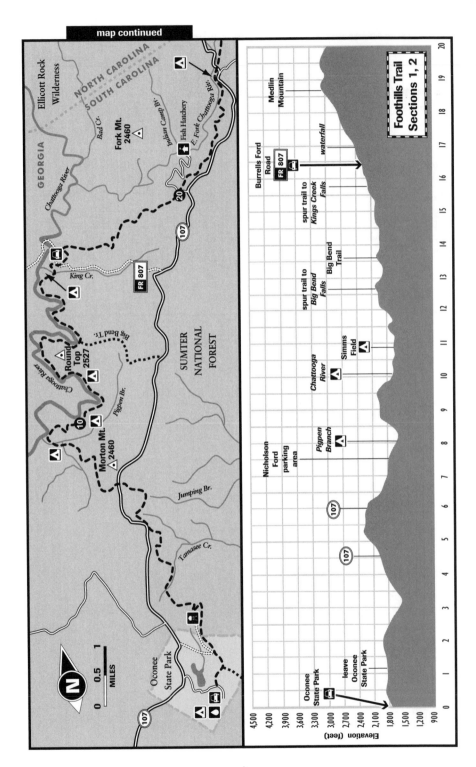

map continued

Ellicott Rock
Wilderness

NORTH CAROLINA
SOUTH CAROLINA

GEORGIA

Chattooga River

Bad Cr.

Fork Mt.
2460

Indian Camp Br.

Fish Hatchery

E. Fork Chattooga Riv.

20

107

King Cr.

FR 807

Big Bend Tr.

Round
Top
2527

Chattooga River

Pigpen Br.

10

Morton Mt.
2460

SUMTER
NATIONAL
FOREST

Jumping Br.

Tamasee Cr.

Oconee
State Park

107

N

0    0.5    1
MILES

**Foothills Trail
Sections 1, 2**

Medlin
Mountain

Burrells Ford
Road

FR 807

waterfall

spur trail to
Kings Creek
Falls

spur trail to
Big Bend
Falls

Big Bend
Trail

Simms
Field

Chattooga
River

Nicholson
Ford
parking
area

Pigpen
Branch

107

107

Oconee
State Park

leave
Oconee
State Park

Elevation (feet)

4,500
4,200
3,900
3,600
3,300
3,000
2,700
2,400
2,100
1,800
1,500
1,200
900

0  1  2  3  4  5  6  7  8  9  10  11  12  13  14  15  16  17  18  19  20

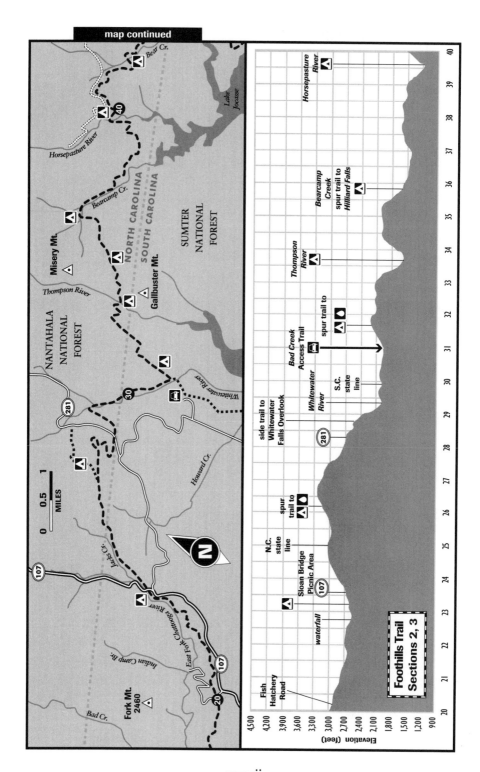

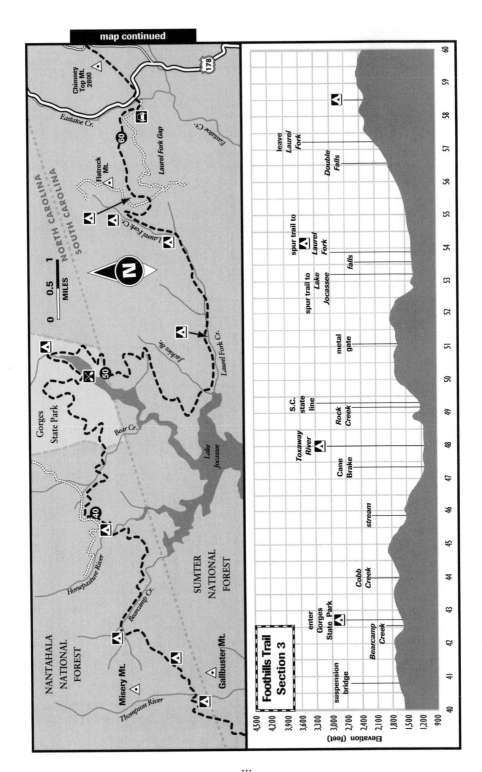

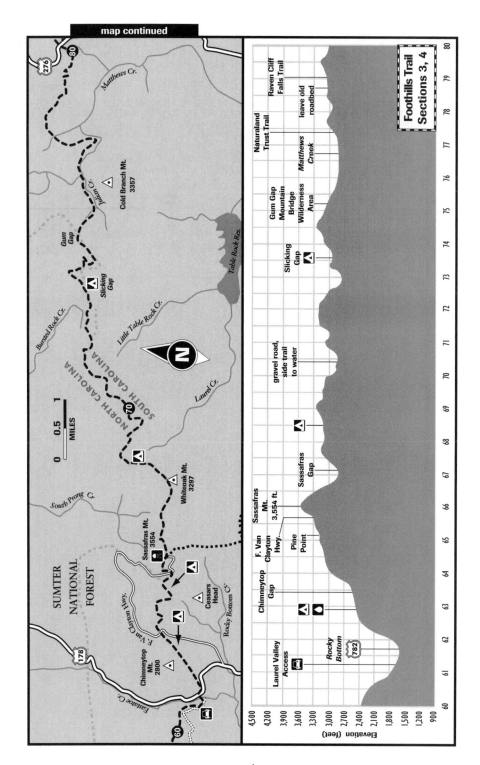

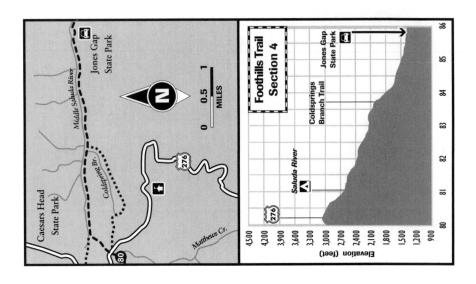

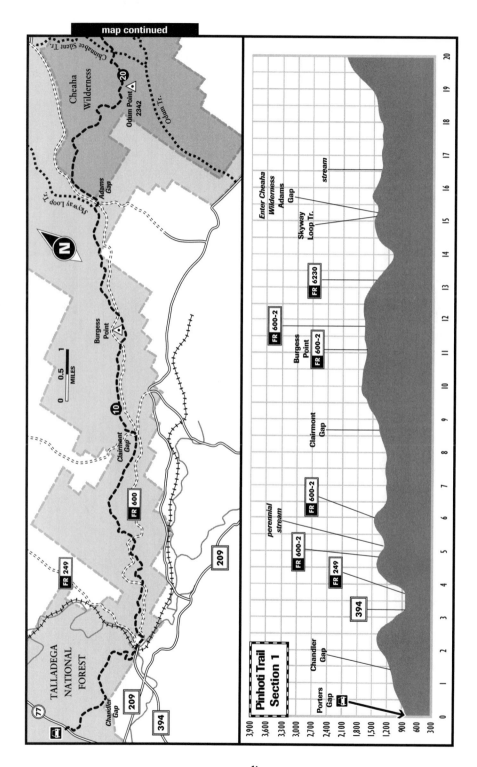

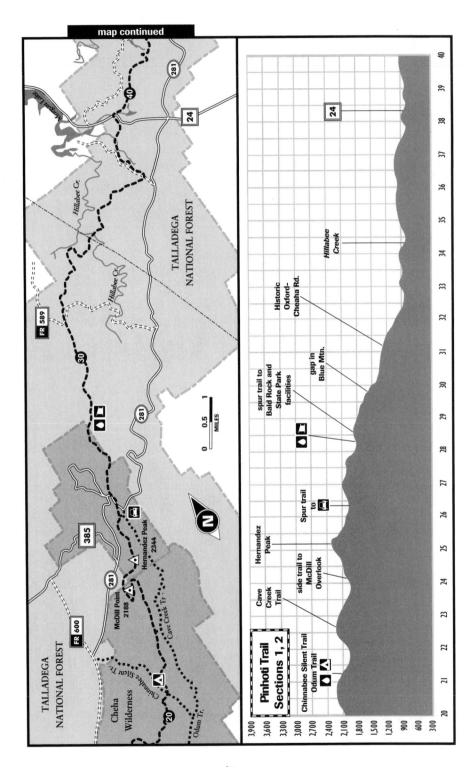

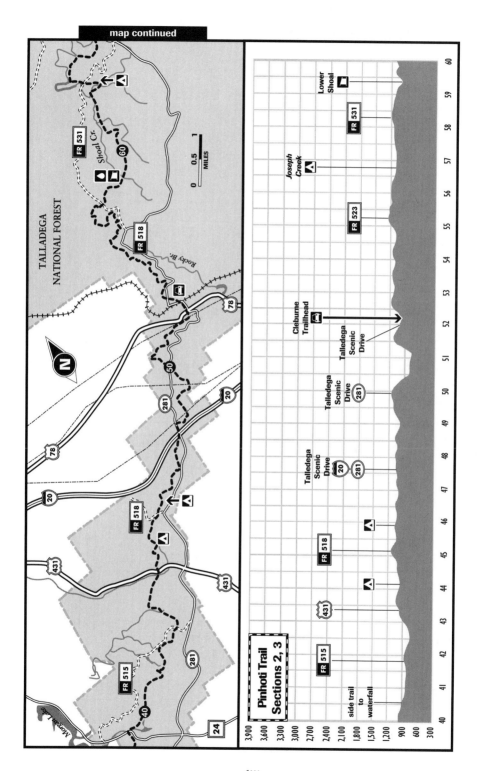

TALLADEGA
NATIONAL FOREST

FR 531

Shoal Cr.

FR 518

Rocky Br.

N

Pinhoti Trail
Sections 2, 3

Lower
Shoal

FR 531

Joseph
Creek

FR 523

Cleburne
Trailhead

Talledega
Scenic
Drive

Talledega
Scenic
Drive

Talledega
Scenic
Drive

FR 518

side trail
to
waterfall

FR 515

MILES

xliii

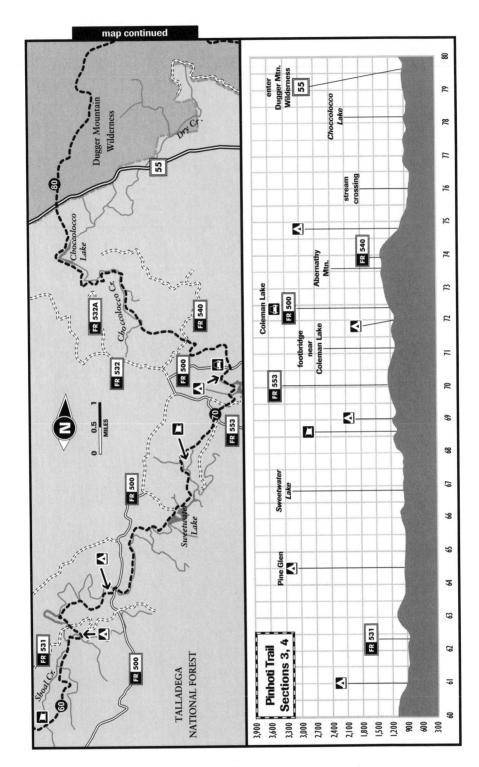

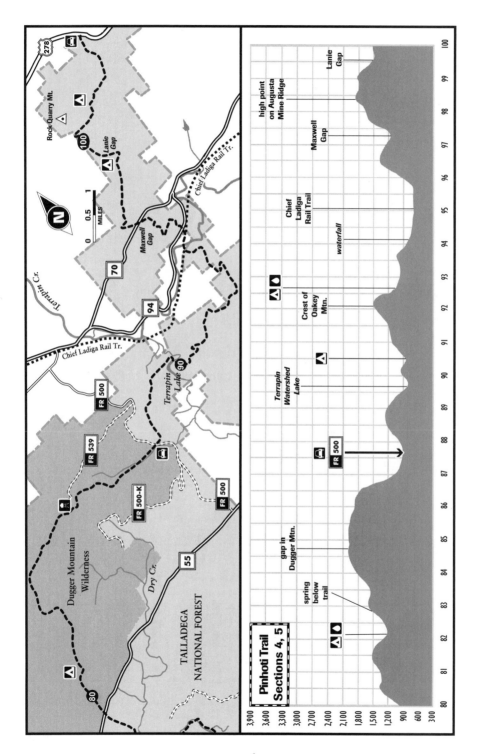

xlv

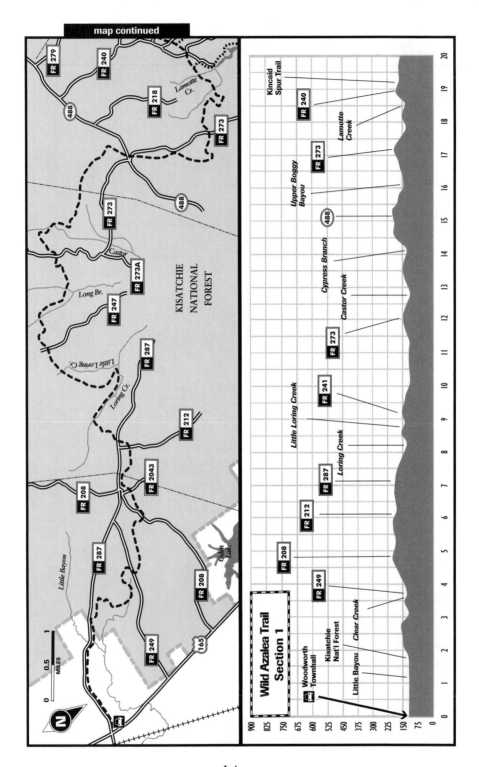

xlvi

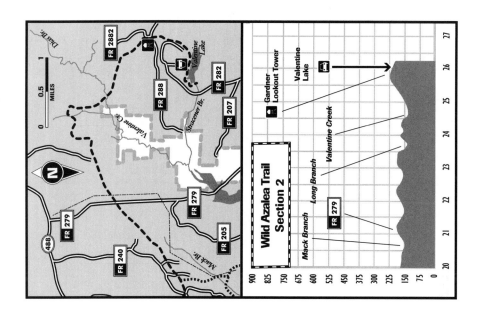

# INTRODUCTION

## A Word about This Book and the Long Trails of the Southeast

In this book you will find over 600 varied miles of long trails to hike, from the cypress swamps of South Florida to the high mountains of North Carolina. Each offers its own beauty and challenges. The Wild Azalea Trail, the shortest of this book's trails at 26 miles, is Louisiana's longest footpath. It will surprise visitors as it rambles over pine-covered hills into lush bottomlands where clear, sand-bottomed streams flow. Wetlands abound in these creek bottoms, locally known as bayous, where the cypress trees grow tall. The 41-mile **Black Creek Trail** of Mississippi runs along the course of the federally designated Wild and Scenic Black Creek, amid cypress swamps, by sugar-white sandbars, and through hardwood forests with amazingly large trees. Seemingly innumerable side creeks feed Black Creek. The trail crosses the feeder streams by boardwalks and footbridges. In other places the path leaves the river and meanders through open pine forests.

Although the **Florida Trail** (FT) is incomplete (it will eventually reach 1,300 miles), I have included three of the longest sections of the trail. The first 42-mile section traverses the Big Cypress National Preserve, where you will be introduced to "swamp slogging" while crossing sawgrass prairies broken by lush tree islands of palm, cypress, and pine. There is simply no other hiking experience in the United States to match it. Farther north, a 60-mile parcel of the FT runs through the Ocala National Forest, where the world's largest tract of sand-pine scrub forest still remains. This ecosystem offers a beauty of its own, along with large, wild lakes, vast prairies, and richly forested islands. The panhandle portion of the Florida Trail through the Apalachicola National Forest is another experience altogether. Here, the 66-mile FT travels through a longleaf pine/wiregrass ecosystem divided by lush forests growing along dark streams. Also expect to see ponds , grassy savannas, and high-banked rivers.

1

Florida's neighbor, "Alabama the beautiful," has the next long trail. Some may chuckle at such a notion, but after hiking the 104-mile **Pinhoti Trail,** you will be singing this tune as well. The Pinhoti follows the most southerly extension of the Appalachian Mountains as it reaches into the Heart of Dixie. To be sure, these mountains may not be as high as others, but they are rugged and offer an allure all their own. Rock-strewn ridges lead to the Cheaha Wilderness where rock outcrops allow you to see to the very end of the mountains and the plains beyond. Farther north is hill and creek country, where hardwood-cloaked slopes lead down to crystal clear streams shaded by beech trees. More views await in the Dugger Mountain Wilderness amid the pines that crown its heights.

Two of the long trails in this book are in Georgia: the **Benton MacKaye Trail** (BMT) and the **Bartram Trail** (BT). The 93-mile Benton MacKaye Trail begins on Springer Mountain, the Appalachian Trail's southern terminus, and heads north along the western rim of the Appalachians. Here it offers views from the Blue Ridge escarpment then descends to span the Toccoa River on an elaborate suspension footbridge. Low, unsung, and little-visited mountains lie ahead before a trek through private property. After reentering National Forest land, the BMT rambles amid some of the most remote lands in the Peach State before making Jacks River and the famed Cohutta Wilderness. The trail enters Tennessee's Cherokee National Forest and the Big Frog Wilderness. Here, the BMT reaches its high point, 4,224 feet, atop Big Frog Mountain before ending near the Ocoee River.

The 110-mile Bartram Trail, named for naturalist William Bartram, offers the longest, continuous trail in the Southeast. The BT starts along the wild and scenic Chattooga River, heading west to reach the stone tower atop Rabun Bald, Georgia's highest foot-accessible-only point. The BT continues north to enter North Carolina and its stone-faced mountains, where views are abundant. A road walk leads across the Little Tennessee River Valley. The Bartram then resumes a path up to the old stone tower on Wayah Bald. Descend to Nantahala Lake and travel along the Nantahala River before reaching Cheoah Bald (5,062 feet).

The 85-mile **Foothills Trail** of South Carolina and North Carolina will stun first-time visitors. It winds through the Cherokee Foothills of the Southern Appalachians. Raise your expectations here, and the

Foothills Trail will meet them. This trail has more incredible waterfalls per mile of trail than any other path I've ever hiked. It also travels along mountaintops, beside wild and scenic rivers, through gorges, across wildernesses, beside a large mountain lake, and into deep forests. An additional 8 miles of hiking could easily hook ambitious hikers up with the previously mentioned Bartram Trail, providing the possibility of 203 miles of uninterrupted hiking.

It is hard to say exactly when, where, or what propelled the development of other long trails in the Southeast besides the Appalachian Trail. The story seems to start in South Carolina, where proud locals recognized all the attractive natural resources they had in their own backyard and pulled private groups and public agencies together to build a "Foothills Trail." The Foothills Trail was begun in 1968 and completed in 1981. Portions of what became the Florida Trail were laid out even earlier, in the mid-1960s, in the Ocala National Forest. Work continues to this day, to complete this orange-blazed path from the Big Cypress Swamp near the Everglades to Santa Rosa Island near Pensacola. The Benton MacKaye Trail was spawned in 1979, for two reasons: to honor Benton MacKaye, the man with the original idea for the Appalachian Trail, and to provide an alternative to the overused Appalachian Trail for getting through northern Georgia and ultimately to the Smoky Mountains. In other areas, National Forest personnel laid out long trails of their own, such as the Black Creek Trail in Mississippi's De Soto National Forest and the Pinhoti Trail of Alabama's Talladega National Forest.

Today a movement is afoot establishing long trails throughout the United States. Some are essentially complete, such as the Pacific Crest Trail. Some are very ambitious and will likely always include road walks, such as the America Discovery Trail, which travels east to west across the United States. But most trails fall into another category, somewhat long, maybe finished, maybe not, such as the Ice Age Trail of Ohio and Wisconsin, the Colorado Trail, West Virginia's Allegheny Trail, Tennessee's Cumberland Trail, or the Sheltowee Trace in Kentucky.

Some trails in this guidebook, such as the Wild Azalea Trail and the Foothills Trail, have set routes. Others are in flux and may be rerouted or extended, such as the Pinhoti and Benton MacKaye. Stay tuned as these long trails of the Southeast continue to evolve over the years to come, adding to the already exciting hiking possibilities.

## How to Use this Guidebook

In this book, each long trail is broken into segments. I divided the long trails into segments to create viable two-, three- or four-day backpacking trips for those wanting to complete a long trail one segment at a time. The segments also appear due to natural divisions in the trail, i.e., one section may be very different from the next. Generally, a hardy hiker can complete each segment in a long weekend.

At the beginning of each segment's introduction is an information box that provides the hiker with quick access to pertinent information: trail segment length, trail condition, highs, lows, season, difficulty, use, and tips. Below is an example of a box included with a trail segment:

# Pinhoti Trail, Porters Gap to Cheaha State Park

| | |
|---|---|
| **Length:** | 26.3 miles |
| **Trail Condition:** | Good |
| **Highs:** | Views, rock outcrops, Cheaha Wilderness |
| **Lows:** | Long dry sections of trail, very rocky path in places |
| **Season:** | Year-round; best during spring and fall, summer can be hot |
| **Difficulty:** | Moderate to difficult |
| **Use:** | Moderate, heavy in Cheaha Wilderness |
| **Tips:** | Start your hike with water and fill up wherever you can, especially in dry times |
| **Campsites:** | 5.1, 13.4, and 21.3 miles |

From the box, readers can discern that the trail segment is 26.3 miles from Porters Gap to Cheaha State Park and that the trail may be faint, rough, or in this case rocky in places. Trailside highs include passing through the Cheaha Wilderness and enjoying views among scattered rock outcrops; trailside lows indicate water is scarce. The trail can be hiked year-round but is best hiked during spring and fall. This segment can be challenging for less-fit hikers. Smart hikers will be filling their water bottles before they start and fill them at water sources whenever they can. Campsites can be found along the trail at 5.1, 13.4, and 21.3 miles.

Following the information box are detailed directions to the trailheads on each end of the segment. Following the directions is a running narrative of the hike. The narrative first gives an overview of the trail segment, followed by a detailed description, including water access locations, campsites and shelters, trail junctions, stream crossings, potential resupply points, and trailside features, along with their distance from the trailhead. These trail features keep you apprised of your whereabouts and give you a heads-up so that you don't miss them.

With seven long trails included in this guide, you could take the whole book along for reference and reading material, or just copy portions of the book that you are hiking, cutting down on pack weight. Either way, the information inside will make for a more informed, better-executed hike.

# LONG TRAILS
# OF THE
# SOUTHEAST

# BARTRAM TRAIL

The Bartram Trail offers the consummate Southern Appalachian experience, as it treks 110 miles from northeast Georgia to western North Carolina through the wooded mountains of Georgia's Chattahoochee National Forest and North Carolina's Nantahala National Forest. Though the Bartram Trail passes through no designated wilderness areas, it certainly exudes a wilderness aura. The path begins along a wild and scenic river, then turns north onto the Blue Ridge, culminating in a 360-degree view from a stone tower atop Rabun Bald. The Bartram Trail travels next into North Carolina amid incredible stone-faced mountains, where the views are all natural. After crossing the Little Tennessee River Valley, the Bartram Trail heads back into the high country, offering another 360-degree view from the old stone tower of Wayah Bald. From here, it's downhill to Nantahala Lake before entering the gorge country of the Nantahala River, topping out with a climb along numerous waterfalls to reach the trail terminus at Cheoah Bald, which functions as a grandstand for the Smoky Mountains.

The Bartram Trail's course, while still being improved, is mostly set. It is well marked, well maintained, and with few exceptions, easy to follow. Quality camping opportunities are many and well spaced from one another, and water access is generally good. Natural features abound from beginning to end, keeping the hiking interesting. However, there is currently a 14-mile road walk stretch through the vicinity of Franklin, North Carolina. A future reroute will eliminate the road walk and possibly shorten the trail. For now, consider the road walk an opportunity for resupply, as it is roughly at the halfway point. Other resupply points are minimal.

The trail is named for eighteenth-century naturalist William Bartram. Inspired by his naturalist father John Bartram, William set out in 1773 to explore the southeastern United States. For four years he cataloged and described the flora, fauna, and American Natives of the region. He is credited with identifying over 200 native plants. His adventure was later published as *Travels of William Bartram*, and is available in bookstores. Bartram's life and contributions still have an impact today—his homeplace and botanical garden is a Philadelphia landmark, and his travels and notes are valuable resources, revealing what much of southeastern America was like more than 200 years ago. Today, the Bartram Trail roughly follows Bartram's journey through the mountains of North Georgia and western North Carolina, attempting to offer a wilderness opportunity reminiscent of Bartram's experience, while promoting further inquiry and knowledge of the Southern Appalachian region.

❀   ❀   ❀

Begin this trek at the Georgia–South Carolina border on the Peach State side of the Chattooga Wild and Scenic River. Follow the yellow diamond-shaped blazes downstream along this Southern treasure, passing old homesites, clear feeder streams, and the rapids of the Chattooga. The well constructed, highly maintained Georgia portion of the Bartram Trail then turns west along a remote rib ridge connecting the Chattooga corridor to the Blue Ridge. Stop by scenic Warwoman Dell, a picnic ground developed by the Civilian Conservation Corps (CCC) back in the 1930s. Ascend past the waterfalls of Martin Creek before turning north along the Blue Ridge, rising ever higher to make Rabun Bald (4,596 feet), the second highest point in Georgia and accessible only by foot. Atop this peak is a stone observation tower, also built by the CCC. The views extend the length of the horizon in all directions, from the Piedmont to the south and east to the stone-sided mountains of North Carolina to the north and west. Catch this view on a clear day and your entire trip will be worthwhile.

Descend into North Carolina, passing small feeder streams along the way. The trail is more rugged in the Tar Heel State, with less evidence of trail maintenance (i. e., tread construction, bridges, and blazes). Furthermore, the blazes here are yellow rectangles instead of diamonds. The Bartram resumes ridge walking to scale Scaly Mountain. The stony face of this peak offers far-reaching views and up-close beauty. Drop into the Tessentee Creek watershed before climbing into the Fishhawk

Mountains, simply one of the most scenic ranges in the country. These ancient highlands have sheer rock sides overlooking the Tessentee Creek Valley. Other parts are clothed in rich woods; others have wildlife clearings that act as mountain meadows. The side trail to the overlook at Whiterock Mountain will stun you, and make you hold on for dear life, as its rockface curves down from its high point for hundreds of feet. More views await on Wolf Rock before the BT drops to Buckeye Creek.

Here begins the road walk, mostly along country lanes, into the town of Franklin, where resupply and overnight lodging are possibilities. Re-enter national-forest land at Wallace Branch. Here, the BT climbs to join Trimont Ridge and wanders through the high country, up and down, ultimately meeting up with the Appalachian Trail near Wayah Bald in the Nantahala Mountains. Wayah Bald features yet another stone tower with views in all directions and an interpretive plaque providing interesting historical information at its peak. Here, the BT and AT travel west together to make Wine Spring Bald, then separate at this point. The Bartram Trail keeps west on McDonald Ridge, leaving the Nantahalas behind. On this spine, the path begins as a wide, pleasant high-country walk, passing through wildlife clearings. Then the ridge narrows to a slim, rocky backbone with steep drops beneath an ever-changing forest to reach Nantahala Lake. A short road walk leads back into the woods, circling around the lake. The BT then turns north below the dam and follows the Nantahala River through private property, eventually rejoining forest land near Appletree Group Camp. The Bartram Trail, which is the master path of the Appletree Trail System, then makes a rugged track along the Nantahala River before turning west, climbing out of the Nantahala Gorge into Poplar Cove. Traverse this small, wild valley to reach the Piercy Creek valley, full of pine trees and everywhere-you-look beauty. Climb away from Piercy Creek to circle around Rattlesnake Knob, from which you can see your ultimate destination, Cheoah Bald.

Once again, drop into the Nantahala Gorge and reach the area that draws outdoor lovers of all stripes. Join a paved greenway and look out on rafters and kayakers plying the nearby fast water of the Nantahala River. Others will be trout fishing and pedaling bicycles. Span the Nantahala on a bridge, then, once again, climb out of the gorge, this time very steeply. Reach Ledbetter Creek, a narrow valley clothed in a northern hardwood forest of yellow birch, beech, and cherry. This quintessential mountain stream falls, tumbles, and cascades in nearly continuous fashion while the Bartram Trail ascends every bit as steeply upward. The BT breaks out of Ledbetter Creek watershed just below Cheoah Bald, where it makes a final climb in conjunction with the Appalachian Trail onto a peak of grassy meadows, trees, and rock outcrops that offer vistas worthy of a trail's end. Look southeast over the mountains through which you walked and northwestward to the Great Smokies.

Camping opportunities along the Bartram Trail are plentiful, with a few exceptions. Backcountry campers must be at least 50 feet from the Chattooga River and its tributaries. Other than that, backcountry camping is allowed anywhere in the Chattahoochee National Forest of Georgia unless specifically prohibited. The same goes for lands in the Nantahala National Forest in North Carolina. However, a few sections of the trail enter private lands, where camping is prohibited. These private lands are easily avoided. Near Nantahala Lake is a private campground that offers showers and even cabins. The real challenge comes on the 14-mile road walk between Buckeye Creek and Wallace Branch. While there is a campground with water about 0.4 miles from the Wallace Branch end of the road walk, the closest water source on the Buckeye Creek end is another 7-mile hike into the woods. Those hikers wanting to camp near water will have a 21-mile hike ahead of them. Hikers may opt to stay in one of several motels half-way along this road walk, or ration water appropriately and camp on either end of the road walk. After the road walk, camping opportunities once again are frequent enough to make extended backpacking easily manageable. Overall, camping is spread among both ridgelines and creeks. Hikers will need to keep apprised of water sources on some of the longer ridge walks.

The Bartram Trail is surprisingly lightly used, with some exceptions. Its beginning portion on the Chattooga River is more heavily walked, as is the area near Rabun Bald. In North Carolina, the Wayah Bald area is busy, as is the paved greenway along the Nantahala River and atop Cheoah Bald. (The Wayah Bald and Cheoah Bald areas run in conjunction with the Appalachian Trail, bringing the crowds.) The entire trail is quiet during winter, but the high elevations on the ridgelines can make an extended winter trip very challenging, with potential for heavy snow and subzero temperatures. The most pleasant times to hike are late spring, summer, and fall. Fall is especially scenic, with clear blue days contrasting with autumn's color parade.

The entire trail can be hiked without resupply, though the Franklin road walk portion avails not only lodging and postal services, but grocery stores and even a laundry. Otherwise, the path passes by one small store with convenience items and limited camping supplies near Nantahala Lake. After hiking the Bartram Trail, your resupply thoughts will probably be geared toward getting enough grub to turn around and do the trail again.

## Bartram Trail, Russell Bridge to Warwoman Dell

| | |
|---|---|
| **Length:** | 18.6 miles |
| **Trail Condition:** | Excellent |
| **Highs:** | Chattooga Wild and Scenic River, Dicks Creek Falls, old homesite, Warwoman Dell Picnic Area |
| **Lows:** | Abused area near Warwoman Ford |
| **Season:** | Year-round |
| **Difficulty:** | Moderate |
| **Use:** | Heavy near Chattooga River, moderate elsewhere |
| **Tips:** | Limited camping last 9 miles of this section |
| **Campsites:** | 1.4, 3.2, 4.3, 6.2, 9.1, and 14.9 miles |

**RUSSELL BRIDGE TRAILHEAD:** From just north of the junction of US 76 and US 441 in Clayton, Georgia, head east on Warwoman Road and follow it 14 miles to intersect GA 28. Turn right on GA 28, and follow it 2.1 miles to the Bartram Trail parking area on your left, just before GA 28 crosses the Chattooga River into South Carolina.

**WARWOMAN DELL TRAILHEAD:** From just north of the junction of US 76 and US 441 in Clayton, Georgia, head east on Warwoman Road and follow it 2.9 miles to Warwoman Dell Picnic Area. Turn right into the picnic area and follow the gravel road 0.2 miles to its end and a parking area.

The southern terminus of the Bartram Trail is also its lowest elevation. Leave the trailhead and travel southwesterly along a beautiful stretch of the federally designated Wild and Scenic Chattooga River. The walking is mostly easy as you head downstream to the lowest elevation of the BT before turning away from the river, passing Dicks Creek Falls. The BT turns west along a ridgeline, leaving the Chattooga watershed behind. Ascend on the ridgeline, reaching a high point near Rainy Mountain before dropping to the headwaters of Warwoman Creek at Warwoman Dell Picnic Area. You will no doubt notice the first of several interesting features of the Bartram Trail's Georgia section—large engraved stone markers of the Bartram Trail, usually located at gaps and roadside trail crossings.

❄    ❄    ❄

A large stone-engraved trail marker lies at the riverside end of the parking area. Start the Bartram Trail by crossing GA 28, away from the parking area and enter the woods, heading downstream along the Chattooga River. Do not take the trail heading north, directly away from the parking area, or the trail running down to the Chattooga parallel to the Highway 28 bridge. The yellow diamond–blazed Bartram Trail follows a single-track path 0.1 miles to intersect an old woods road. Keep forward down the woods road, passing the concrete abutments of an old bridge to reach a long footbridge spanning the West Fork of the Chattooga River. Walk over the bridge, looking down on the sand-bottomed West Fork and left to the confluence of the West Fork and Chattooga rivers. Turn left after the bridge and cruise through pine woods. The BT straddles the floodplain to your left and the hillside to your right. Campsites are scattered in the pines below. Be apprised, cars are audible from SC 28 across the river.

Return to the Chattooga. Old roads spoke outward, but the main path is evident. Disturbed areas are grown up in tulip trees. Kudzu adds a brushy element to the trailside scenery. At mile 1.2, span Holden Creek on a footbridge. The BT turns right just past the bridge, ascending steps.

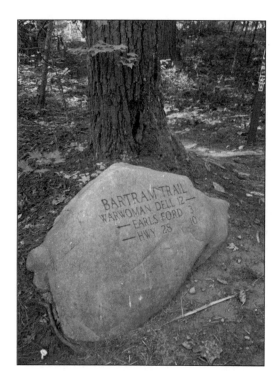

Stone-engraved trail marker

Rejoin an old roadbed flanked by mountain laurel. At mile 1.4, a boat launch off SC 28 is visible to your left through the trees. Shortly, pass through a campsite, then span a small stream on a footbridge. Holly trees are scattered in the flat. An old barbed wire fence indicates former farmland.

Shortly, pass an old metal hay baler on trail-left. Several old roads converge here. Just after a boardwalk spanning a shallow branch, look right for a standing old stone chimney that was once someone's hearth. To your left is a white pine copse. The BT keeps forward through the large flat before diverging right at mile 2.2 to rise over a low ridge. Intersect an orange diamond–marked horse trail at mile 2.5. Turn right, walk just a short distance, then veer back left. Descend to reach a flat stretch on Adline Branch. Bridge the creek in a thicket of holly trees. A campsite lies beneath pine and hemlock trees near the stream. Ascend away from Adline Branch on a single-track footpath passing through pine-oak woods. Top a hill and descend through mountain laurel to reach Bynum

Branch at mile 3.2. Span this creek on a bridge and pass another camp-site on the left. Ascend again, topping out at mile 3.6. The BT runs in conjunction with a horse trail just a short distance then makes an acute right turn, descending a dry draw. Circle the hillside to span Laurel Branch in a dark rhododendron thicket at mile 4.1. Parallel the branch beneath hemlock trees. Meanwhile, the Chattooga River is making a long bend to the south. The forest changes instantly to oak as the BT tops a hill and drops to a bridge that crosses a small, unnamed stream. A small, sloped campsite lies just after the bridge at mile 4.3.

Ascend away from this stream and join an old road, making a sharp left turn onto a single-track path at mile 4.7. The pine-oak woods once again give way to rhododendron along a small stream with a footbridge at mile 5.0. Work around the south side of Willis Knob before intersect-ing a wide, road-like horse trail at mile 5.9. Keep forward, descending along a hollow rife with ferns to near Warwoman Creek, which is down to the right. A faint side trail leads acutely right to a campsite on this creek. Parallel Warwoman Creek, heading downstream before turning right at a metal footbridge spanning the clear watercourse at mile 6.3. Continue downstream just after the bridge beneath towering white pines along Warwoman Creek. Soon enough, the auto accessibility of War-woman Ford degrades the area. Cross the gravel Earls Ford Road at mile 6.5. The actual Earls Ford is on the Chattooga. Pass through beat-up campsites along Warwoman Creek in a large flat. Cross a wooden bridge standing 10 feet over a small streamlet flowing into Warwoman Creek. The large waterside flat ends. Leave Warwoman Creek for good at mile 7.1. The BT leaves right off of an old road as single-track footpath, meandering through laurel-oak woods above a gap to your left. Rejoin the old road before returning to a hemlock flat on the Chattooga River at mile 7.8. Soon, pass a grassy vista of the river before spanning a small gullied creek on a footbridge. Several campsites lie near the river.

At mile 8.3, turn away from the Chattooga for good onto an ascend-ing single-track path. Bisect a small gap before descending to span a streamlet. Keep downstream, passing some well-used campsites before coming to a trail junction at mile 9.1. To your left, a side trail spans the small stream and heads on a short piece to the top of Dicks Creek Falls, a 60-foot cascade with a view of the Chattooga to boot. To the right, an old road heads uphill toward private land and Antioch, Georgia. The BT continues forward to span Dicks Creek on a wooden bridge. Just to the right before the Dicks Creek bridge is a side trail to a level campsite. Dicks Creek is the last easy water access for 6 miles.

The BT now runs along Dicks Creek, ascending steps, then reaches a trail junction and stone-engraved trail marker at mile 9.4. The Chattooga Trail, with silver diamond blazes, keeps left and heads downriver to the US 76 bridge. The yellow-blazed BT keeps right, uphill, to reach Sandy Ford Road at mile 9.5. Cross the dirt road and keep uphill, passing another stone-engraved trail marker. Switchback uphill in pine-oak woods on a single-track path, picking up a westward-leading ridgeline roughly paralleling Dicks Creek. Watch for mica rock shimmering on the trailbed at your feet. At mile 10.1, pick up a woods road in a gap, where five old roads come together. Stay with the yellow blazes, as the BT shortly resumes single-track. Work along the steepening north side of the ridgeline, spanning a dry streambed on a footbridge at mile 11.0. Descend to reach Speed Gap at mile 11.4, marked by a carved stone marker. In the gap, a view is open to the south. Leave the gap on a single-track path, avoiding the old roads. Ascend west on the ridgeline, then pick up an old road. Briefly leave the road at mile 11.9. To your left are the knobs of Rainy Ridge, where the Bartram Trail leads.

Undulate along the ridgeline in mostly pine woods, complemented with sourwood. Drop steeply to reach Bob Gap, also marked with a carved stone, at mile 12.9. Cross gravel Pool Ridge Road at the gap and climb, reaching the ridgeline and a woods road at mile 13.3, in a forest of maple, sourwood, and pine. Continue climbing over knobs east of Rainy Mountain. Some places are quite steep. At mile 14.7, on an ascent out of a gap, leave the old roadbed, turning sharply right onto a single-track path. Skirt around to the north side of the Rainy Mountain, passing a small, crummy campsite on a rib ridge at mile 14.9, before descending into a rhododendron thicket and a spring branch at mile 15.1. You will probably have to work under the rhododendron upstream to reach water falling over a small rockface.

Turn north on Rainy Ridge among mountain laurel. At mile 15.9, reach the crest of Rainy Ridge. A red-blazed side trail leads left up the nose of the ridge. Keep north, and watch for the yellow blazes, as the BT makes an abrupt and unexpected right turn off a woods road at mile 16.1. Drift on and off the ridgeline, reaching a trail junction at mile 17.0.

A trail blazed with silver-colored goat figures intersects from the left. The "Goat Trail" and Bartram Trail run in conjunction downhill in pine-laurel woods to reach Green Gap and an inscripted rock at mile 17.3. Here, the "Goat Trail" leaves left, while the BT ascends steeply from Green Gap in rocky woods, leveling off on the ridgeline. At mile 17.7, gain a southward view of Lake Toccoa in the immediate valley below and the state of Georgia as far as the sky allows. Drop off the ridgeline, keeping on a single-track path, crossing three tiny streamsheds on wooden footbridges before reaching Warwoman Dell Picnic Area at mile 18.6. This attractive setting has a covered picnic shelter, rest room, and water spigot. The spigot is about 20 feet to the left of the picnic shelter and runs during the warm season. A trailside kiosk tells of the attempt to develop the Blue Ridge Railroad, connecting Charleston, South Carolina, with Cincinnati, Ohio, via Knoxville, Tennessee. The project was ultimately undone by the coming of the Civil War. The picnic area marks the end of this section of the Bartram Trail. Camping is not allowed in the picnic area. However, campsites with water are 2 miles distant along Martins Creek.

# Bartram Trail, Warwoman Dell to Hale Ridge Road

| | |
|---|---|
| **Length:** | 17.7 miles |
| **Trail Condition:** | Excellent |
| **Highs:** | Becky Falls, Martin Creek Falls, view from Flat Top, 360-degree view from Rabun Bald |
| **Lows:** | Trail approaches houses near Beegum Gap |
| **Season:** | Year-round, Rabun Bald area could be very cold in winter |
| **Difficulty:** | Moderate to difficult, first 13 miles mostly uphill |
| **Use:** | Heavy near Rabun Bald, a little less busy near Warwoman Dell, moderate elsewhere |
| **Tips:** | Be apprised of water supplies, though occasional sources are located throughout section |
| **Campsites:** | 2.0, 5.0, 11.8, 16.5, and 17.5 miles |

**WARWOMAN DELL TRAILHEAD:** From just north of the junction of US 76 and US 441 in Clayton, Georgia, head east on Warwoman Road and follow it 2.9 miles to Warwoman Dell Picnic Area. Turn right into the picnic area and follow the gravel road 0.2 miles to its end and a parking area.

**HALE RIDGE ROAD TRAILHEAD:** From Dillard, Georgia, on US 441, 0.7 miles south of the North Carolina state line, take GA 246 east for 4 miles to Old Mud Creek Road. Turn right onto Old Mud Creek Road, which becomes Bald Mountain Road. Go 4 miles to Hale Ridge Road. Turn right onto Hale Ridge Road and follow it for 1.1 miles. The road becomes gravel 0.3 miles before reaching the trailhead, which will be on your left. The parking area is on the right. Park beyond the first sign for the Bartram Trail, indicating Rabun Bald. A larger parking area is around the corner past this sign.

This section steadily and surely heads into the high country, capping out in a vista from an open wooden platform atop Rabun Bald, before descending past many streamlets to reach Hale Ridge Road just shy of the North Carolina state line. Pass waterfalls near the section's beginning, picking up the Blue Ridge. Traverse over and around knobs divided by gaps. After making it to the top of Rabun Bald, the climbing moderates, and the walking is easy.

Campsites with water are limited in this section. Martin Creek offers quality camping, as does a high but small spot near Flat Top, with its great views. A prescribed burn area beyond Flat Top offers insight into fire ecology and forest progression after such fires. The BT passes near the national-forest boundary after Rabun Bald, nearing mountain homes before cruising along a slope east of Ford Mountain. Limited, small campsites are near some small streams emanating from Ford Mountain.

❂    ❂    ❂

Leave the parking area beside the covered picnic shelter at the rear of Warwoman Dell. Backtrack down the picnic area road. The BT leaves left from the gravel road just before an information kiosk describing the old fish hatchery that was constructed between 1933–37. Walk just a few feet beyond the turn and inspect the old rearing tanks, once full of feisty trout. Return to the BT and ascend along Becky Branch, shortly reaching

Warwoman Road at 0.2 miles. Pass a roadside metal plaque commemorating William Bartram just before crossing Warwoman Road. Enter the woods and the Warwoman Wildlife Management Area, climbing sharply along Becky Branch and soon reaching Becky Branch Falls. The trail splits beyond the cascade—the right fork returns to Warwoman Dell. The BT stays left to enter an area burned by fire. The trail acted as a firebreak at this point, but further ahead, the fire jumped the trail; evidence of fire can be seen on both sides of the path. The broken woods avail views toward an unnamed knob near Warwoman Dell. At 0.5 miles, bisect a bulldozed firebreak heading straight up the forested ridgeline, spared from fire's destruction by the firebreak.

The BT parallels Warwoman Road below. Span a footbridge over a streamlet at mile 1.0, before turning north into the Finney Creek valley in maple-pine-laurel woods. At mile 1.8, the single-track path merges left onto an old woods road. Martin Creek, a feeder branch of Finney Creek, crashes below, shooting through a mini-gorge. The trail reaches a camping flat across Martin Creek at mile 2.0. Ahead are more campsites in hemlock and white pines. At mile 2.1, a side trail leads right over a wooden bridge and makes a short loop, passing a rock house before reaching Martin Creek Falls, a two-tiered cascade framed in rhododendron. The BT soon leaves the flat, turns left up a small side branch, then picks up a woods road, climbing to near the top of Martin Creek Falls. Resume the single-track path and ascend into an oak forest. Pass a small branch and small campsite, then resume ascending, dipping in and out of hollows. Raven Knob and Wild Hog Ridge stand across the Martin Creek valley.

Begin circling the upper watershed of Martin Creek. Reach a trail junction at mile 3.5 after spanning a stream on a footbridge. To your left, a white-blazed trail follows a jeep road to Pinnacle Knob and a rocky vista. The BT picks up the same roadbed and leaves right to reach Courthouse Gap at mile 3.8. Here, the white-blazed trail leads left and the BT heads forward, up the ominous looking Hogback. The path does climb sharply, but then reaches a roadbed angling uphill around the east side of Hogback. Join the Tennessee Valley Divide near a gap between Hogback and Raven Knob at mile 4.1 and resume the climb. At mile 5.0, cross a tiny streamlet in a hollow. Uphill and to your left as you face the streamlet is a small campsite situated on an old roadbed, the only level spot around. At mile 5.3, reach a rocky gap north of Raven Knob. This flat is much larger, but for camping you have to haul your water from the previous streamlet.

Climb by switchbacks through an attractive open hardwood forest on Rock Mountain, breaking the 3,000-foot mark along the way. At mile 6.2, pick up an obvious roadbed and begin swinging around the northwest side of the Rock Mountain. Keep a nearly level course through rhododendron before dropping to Windy Gap and an inscribed stone at mile 7.1. Ascend out of Windy Gap, grabbing occasional views to the southeast and work along the east side of Black Knob, crossing a pair of small streams at mile 8.0. Leave the streamshed, cruising through a wide-open hardwood forest before arriving at Wilson Gap and an inscribed stone at mile 8.5. Gravel FR 155 passes through the gap. Keep forward, ascending on the forest road for half a mile, looking left for another inscribed stone. At the stone, follow the BT left, leaving the forest road behind. Continue to follow an incline up and around the west side of Double Knob, with far-reaching views to the north and west. Below lie Ramey Field and obviously logged forests of different ages. Across Ramey Creek is the rockface of Flat Top, where the BT soon leads.

Keep north below Wilson Knob. At mile 10.2, reach a gap between Wilson Knob and Flat Top. The dry campsite here has a horizontal rock slab located beneath an open canopy. Continue up the switchbacks, and at the eighth switchback, catch your breath and enjoy a southern view of mountains fading into the Piedmont. Beyond the switchbacks, at mile 10.5, look left for a side trail leading left to a fantastic view from a rockface. Here, the horizon stretches southward from east to west. The BT leads beyond the vista to a spring creek running beneath laurel and rhododendron with an overstory of oak. A small but level campsite lies on the far side of the spring creek.

Pass through a prescribed burn area. Notice the regenerating chestnut, oak, and pine. Views are numerous in the uncanopied spots as the trail switchbacks up, then back down to reach Saltrock Gap. Continue through the wide gap to a split in the trail at mile 11.8. Here, the BT leaves sharply right, and an obvious roadbed keeps forward into rhododendron to shortly reach water, making Saltrock Gap a viable camping spot. The BT follows switchbacks uphill, where a tiny spring crosses the trail at mile 12.3. Keep ascending to reach Flint Gap and a junction with

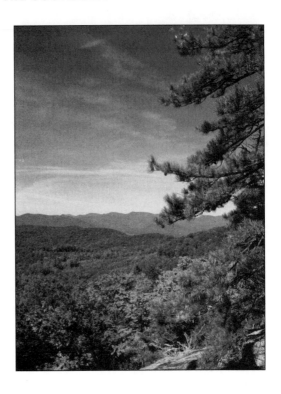

View from Flat Top

an unnamed trail at mile 12.7. An inscribed rock marks the spot. To the left, a blue-blazed trail leads toward Flint Knob.

The BT keeps forward, then turns right and begins switchback after switchback, ascending the west side of Rabun Bald through mountain laurel, oak, and birch. Top out on the knife-edge crest of the ridge, reaching the top of Rabun Bald and an inscribed rock at mile 13.5. Uphill to the right is the stone viewing tower. Climb the tower to a wooden platform and look out in all directions. To the west are the towns in the Little Tennessee River Valley. To the north stand the stony faced mountains of North Carolina. To the east are the Cherokee Foothills of South Carolina and the Piedmont beyond. To the south are the North Georgia Mountains and the Piedmont in the distance. The Three Forks Trail mentioned on the inscribed rock is now called the Rabun Bald Trail, and leaves right 3 miles to Hale Ridge Road.

The BT continues north, descending from Rabun Bald on a rocky tread through a low oak forest. Oddly enough, you pass four low, stone dams crossing the trail. Reach a junction at mile 14.2. A rough road leads left to Beegum Gap. The BT veers right and keeps descending along a gullied old road. Birch and a few cherry trees appear on this north-facing slope. At mile 14.9, after a sharp right turn, the BT keeps forward and leaves the roadbed that heads left toward Beegum Gap. This single-track trail passes over a flat and bisects a dirt road at mile 15.1., which leads left to a house within sight of the trail. Start descending to reach a clear mountain stream spanned by two small wooden bridges connected by a small island at mile 15.6. These are the first two, of eight, bridges spanning perennial and intermittent streams in the next half mile. Beyond the last crossing, pass a rock slab in the woods at mile 16.3. Span another branch on a bridge at mile 16.5, then step over an old road. Downhill to the right is a potential but unlevel campsite. Climb away from the stream, passing through a white pine grove. Descend to a curved bridge below a low-flow waterfall spilling over a wide rockface at mile 17.2. At the third bridge past this waterfall, on your right at mile 17.5, is a small, but level campsite. However, Hale Ridge Road is nearby and auto noise is audible. From here, the BT crosses one last bridge then emerges onto Hale Ridge Road. Turn right and walk down gravel Hale Ridge Road a short piece to reach a signboard beside the BT continuing left into the woods and the end of this section at mile 17.7.

# Bartram Trail, Hale Ridge Road to Buckeye Creek

| | |
|---|---|
| **Length:** | 19.0 miles |
| **Trail Condition:** | Good |
| **Highs:** | View from Scaly Mountain, numerous vistas in Fishhawk Mountains, solitude |
| **Lows:** | Limited campsites with water |
| **Season:** | Year-round |
| **Difficulty:** | Moderate to difficult, many ups and downs |
| **Use:** | Almost all moderate, busier around Jones Gap |
| **Tips:** | Choose your campsites wisely, planning for upcoming 14-mile road walk across Little Tennessee River valley and Franklin |
| **Campsites:** | 1.5, 3.0, 8.0, and 12.1 miles |

**HALE RIDGE ROAD TRAILHEAD:** From Dillard, Georgia, on US 441, 0.7 miles south of the North Carolina state line, take GA 246 east for 4 miles to Old Mud Creek Road. Turn right onto Old Mud Creek Road, which becomes Bald Mountain Road, for 4 miles to Hale Ridge Road. Turn right onto Hale Ridge Road and follow it for 1.1 miles. The road becomes gravel 0.3 miles before reaching the trailhead, which will be on your left. The parking area is on the right. Park beyond the first sign for the Bartram Trail, indicating Rabun Bald. A larger parking area is around the corner past this sign.

**BUCKEYE CREEK TRAILHEAD:** From Franklin, North Carolina, at the point where US 64 and US 441 intersect, head south on US 441 for 7.9 miles to Tessentee Road (SR 1636). Turn left on Tessentee Road, and follow it 3.8 miles to gravel Buckeye Branch Road (SR 1640). Turn left onto Buckeye Branch Road and follow it 0.5 miles to a dead end at a parking area on your right. The Bartram Trail passes directly along this road.

This section of the Bartram Trail is underused relative to its outstanding features. Head north from Hale Ridge Road, shortly entering North Carolina and the Nantahala National Forest. Before ascending Scaly Mountain, travel the seldom-visited Overflow Creek Backcountry Area near Osage Mountain. Here, the rocky crest of this peak offers scenic, far-reaching views. Keep north, descending to Tessentee Creek and a campsite with water, one of the few in this section. Climb again to the high country and the Fishhawk Mountains, where the rocky summits offer exhilarating vistas from stone slabs covering vast sections of mountainside. Descend from the Fishhawks to reach the Buckeye Creek trailhead.

Campsites and water are limited, so plan accordingly. The biggest challenge is camping toward the end of this section. The last site with water, Whiterock Gap, is 7 miles back from the Buckeye Creek trailhead. Hikers proceeding to the next section face a 21-mile hike (14 of this is a road walk) if they want to camp were water is available. Otherwise, take a break and stay at one of the hotels along the way, or make sure you top off those water bottles in Franklin.

Start this section of the Bartram Trail by heading north from Hale Ridge Road, passing a trail information board. The BT enters the woods and ascends, following both yellow rectangular blazes and yellow diamond blazes. Soon bisect an old road. At this location the yellow diamond blazes end, signifying the end of the Georgia portion of the BT. Stay with the rectangular yellow blazes as you enter North Carolina and the Nantahala National Forest. Shortly, cross a small stream on a board bridge passing through rhododendron, ascending the east flank of Osage Mountain on a footpath. Rise then curve left toward a gap at 0.9 miles. Continue in a pine-oak forest broken with pockets of rhododendron in moist hollows. Small streams flow from these hollows and form the headwaters of Web Branch, which feeds Overflow Creek and ultimately the Chattooga River. At mile 1.5, after a seep, look for a small campsite on an old roadbed below to your right. Keep forward, spanning a couple of more streambeds on hewn-log bridges. These bridges are a preferable and rustic contrast to the more elaborate wooden footbridges of the Georgia portion of the Bartram Trail.

Intersect the Hurrah Ridge Trail at mile 2.6. It leads right 0.6 miles to FR 79 and the West Fork Trail. The BT veers left and reaches the

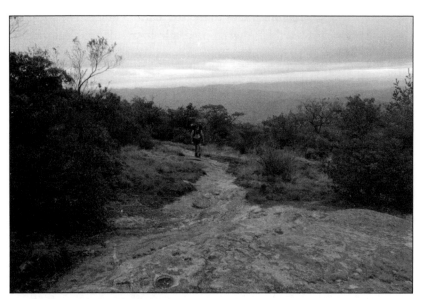

The author headed up Scaly Mountain

3,400-foot level around West Fork Overflow Creek. Yellow birch trees, which are more typical of northern hardwood forests, begin to appear. At mile 3.0, intersect the West Fork Trail just after crossing two log bridges spanning the headwaters of West Fork Overflow Creek. A small campsite lies at this junction. The West Fork Trail veers right 1 mile to FR 79. The BT ascends away from the junction as a single-track path. Shortly, squeeze under a boulder forming a small overhang. At mile 3.2, the BT turns acutely left, while a blue-blazed side trail heads up to Osage Mountain Overlook at NC 106. The BT climbs along a rhododendron-choked streamlet. Meet the blue-blazed side trail again just before reaching the Osage Mountain Overlook and NC 106 at mile 3.6. Cross the paved highway, re-enter the woods, climb steps, and then pass a stone sign that reads, "Constructed By The U.S. Youth Conservation Corps 1980." Ascend steadily in a young forest on the corps-constructed trail. At mile 3.9, a side trail leads left to a small waterfall. The BT keeps forward and shortly crosses the stream above the waterfall. Ascend Scaly Mountain by switchbacks among sporadic rhododendron thickets. Gain glimpses of Scaly Mountain's rockface. At mile 4.5, turn sharply right onto a roadbed. To the left are houses just outside the nearby national-forest border. Turn right and keep climbing the rocky woods road. The BT soon offers far-reaching views to the south as it climbs. The tower of Rabun Bald is easily visible. Ahead, look right for a side trail leading to a wide rockface open to the south. Walk around this rockface to gain more views.

Beyond the rockface, the BT becomes one with a spring seep. Laurel, brush, and low-slung trees flank the trail, which is open to the sky. At mile 5.0, the BT turns sharply left. A blue-blazed side trail leads right, down to Hickory Knut Road. The BT ascends, passing by rockfaces with wide-ranging views. At mile 5.5, top-out your ascent at 4,804 feet atop Scaly Mountain. Begin descending among low-slung oaks and ancient, thick-trunked mountain laurel. Pass another rockface offering westerly views before reaching Gall Tree Gap in a laurel thicket at mile 5.9. Turn right here and keep dropping, now by switchbacks on a single-track path among mountain laurel with massive bases. The descent moderates at mile 6.6, as the BT cruises along the ridgetop. Pines become more prevalent. Soon, resume the switchbacks, criss-crossing a faint roadbed between Tessentee Creek and one of its feeder branches. Make one last super-steep drop just before the two creek's confluence. Span the feeder stream on a wooden bridge and reach the Tessentee Creek campsite at mile 8.0. The camping area lies in hemlocks and yellow birch beside a grassy clearing. Even if you don't camp here, get water here. This is the last water that crosses the trail for 11 miles. (Water is accessible at 4.0 and 4.5 miles distant, but you must leave the BT to access it.)

Turning right, join a wide roadbed beyond the campsite. Do not cross Tessentee Creek. Pass by the clearing and walk the wide roadbed for 0.3 miles to where the BT leaves the road and turns acutely right, up log steps on a single-track path. Negotiate a switchback, then traverse the rough terrain west of Peggy Knob. The going is slow here, as the trail twists and turns among big boulders on a steep slope. An outcrop provides fine views of the Tessentee Creek Valley and the rockfaces of the Fishhawk Mountains ahead. The BT eases up beyond a small knob at mile 9.3. The trail now circles into a deep hollow, then switchbacks out of the hollow to intersect a dirt road at mile 9.7. Turn right on the road and walk just a few feet. Ahead and uphill of you is private property; turn left, and follow the single-track path. Reach the ridgecrest at mile 9.9, joining the Fishhawk Mountains at the 4,000-foot mark. Keep ascending among large oak trees, opening to a rockface with east facing views. At mile 10.3, a short side trail leads left to a direct view of Peggy Knob. Merge onto an old roadbed and top out on Keith Day Knob. Descend from the knob into a wildlife clearing, then through spindly woods before passing around a metal forest service gate and reaching Jones Gap at mile 10.8. Here is a parking area and trail information board at the end of FR 4522.

At Jones Gap, bisect the gravel parking area and pass around a second metal gate. Trace a grassy lane flanked with fire cherry and locust trees, indicating recent reforestation. Reach the far side of a narrow wildlife clearing at mile 11.1. At the far end of the clearing, a blue-blazed side trail leads left 0.3 miles to the top of Jones Knob. This side trail is well worth the effort. From atop Jones Knob, you can overlook the Tessentee Creek Valley and the striated white markings on the face of Whiterock Mountain next door. Continuing past the side trail, the BT skirts around the east side of Jones Knob, winding among rocks, moss, and rhododendron with a hardwood and hemlock overstory. Regain the ridgecrest at mile 11.9. Just ahead, a side trail leads left to a rockface and views. Descend just a bit more to reach Whiterock Gap at mile 12.1. A wooden sign announces the elevation as 4,150 feet. A level but potentially windblown campsite is located here. A spur trail to the right leads 800 feet down to Stevens Creek.

The BT leaves Whiterock Gap, ascending along the east side of Whiterock Mountain. At mile 12.5, a side trail leads right a short distance to a spring. This is the last water for the next 6 miles; get water here if you didn't get it at Whiterock Gap. After a small climb, reach the blue-blazed side trail leading left 0.3 miles to a vista on Whiterock Mountain. This side trail climbs over the top of the mountain, passing several rockfaces, then descends to reach the granddaddy rockface of them all, which drops for hundreds of uninterrupted feet toward Tessentee Creek Valley. The Bartram Trail veers right and keeps climbing in thick woods, crossing occasional rockfaces, some with views. Piled rocks, or cairns, occasionally mark the path across these slabs of stone.

Begin switchbacking up the south side of Little Fishhawk Mountain, peaking out at mile 13.1, near the actual high point of the mountain. Continue downhill, still on a single-track path. Pass through rhododendron thickets before reaching a gap between Little Fishhawk and Fishhawk Mountains. Ascend just a bit before intersecting a side trail leading right to the top of Fishhawk Mountain at mile 13.6. This little-used side trail rises steeply for 0.3 miles, not 300 feet as the trail sign states. At the top you'll find a plaque memorializing William Bartram.

The BT keeps forward, curving around the west side of Fishhawk Mountain, through low boulders and tunnels of rhododendron on a rough tread to reach a tiny gap between Fishhawk Mountain and Wolf Rock at mile 14.5. Striped maple and white birch are prevalent in damper areas. Keep north on a knife-edge ridge. Franklin is visible through the trees to your right. Reach Wolf Rock Overlook, an excellent vista, at mile 15.0. Continue on the narrow ridge spine and switchback near a rockface just below the overlook. The BT has now turned west, as it makes more switchbacks, then narrows to reach a gap at mile 15.6. An old roadbed bisects the gap. Keep forward, ascending a bit, then work along a dramatic wooded bluffline with more views. Wind in and out of thin soiled woods broken by rock outcrops and flat rockfaces. Oddly

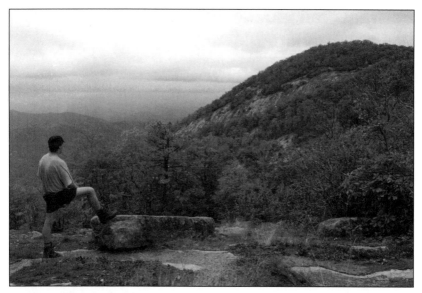

Looking at Whiterock Mountain

enough, on the national-forest boundary line, pass by an old school bus at mile 16.3. It was once part of a now-abandoned hunter's camp. How it got here is lost to time. Pass by the left side of the bus and descend by more views to reach a gap at mile 16.7. Here, the BT leaves the Fishhawk Mountains and turns acutely left toward Buckeye Creek. Cedar Cliff is just ahead. The relatively large gap just above the turn is suitable for camping. However, no water is available nearby. A huge oak tree stands in this gap.

Descend into the Buckeye Creek watershed. Tulip trees dominate the forest. Pick up an old roadbed growing up with young trees just before crossing an intermittent streambed at mile 17.5. This roadbed leads to a second rocky roadbed of red clay at mile 17.7. Turn right on the second roadbed and keep dropping to reach a flowing stream at mile 17.9. The branch flows down a rockface then under the roadbed via a culvert. Make a pleasant forest cruise through coves of tulip trees and un-canopied woods of pine and oak. Span a final tiny creek by culvert at mile 18.7, before reaching a forest service gate at mile 19.0. Walk a bit down the gravel road to reach the Bartram Trail parking area to your left and the end of this section.

# Bartram Trail, Buckeye Creek to Wallace Branch

| | |
|---|---|
| **Length:** | 14.2 miles |
| **Trail Condition:** | Good, all roads |
| **Highs:** | Resupply, lodging, and laundry opportunities |
| **Lows:** | Entire section is a road walk |
| **Season:** | Year-round; could be hot during height of summer |
| **Difficulty:** | Easy on the lungs, hard on the feet |
| **Use:** | Minimal, walked only by end-to-end hikers |
| **Tips:** | Must plan your camping here, either with lodging in Franklin or traversing the entire 14-mile road walk |

**BUCKEYE CREEK TRAILHEAD:** From Franklin, at the point where US 64 and US 441 cross, head south on US 441 for 7.9 miles to Tessentee Road (SR 1636). Turn left on Tessentee Road, and follow it 3.8 miles to gravel Buckeye Branch Road (SR 1640). Turn left onto Buckeye Branch Road and follow it 0.5 miles to a dead end at a parking area on your right. The Bartram Trail passes right along this road.

**WALLACE BRANCH TRAILHEAD:** From the Wayah Ranger Station in Franklin, head north on Sloan Road just a short distance to Old Murphy Road. Cross Old Murphy Road to reach Pressley Road. Keep forward on Pressley Road for 1.7 miles to reach the Wallace Branch trailhead. Do not be tempted to turn left onto Wallace Branch Road. It does not lead to the trailhead. The Bartram Trail road walk ends at the rear of the parking area, immediately spanning a wooden bridge over Wallace Branch.

After traversing the Chattooga River, Rabun Bald, Scaly Mountain, and the Fishhawk Mountains, this section is bound to be a disappointment. The entire section is a road walk, albeit mostly on secondary country roads. Most section hikers will probably opt to avoid this section, but end-to-end hikers have little choice. To connect the Fishhawk Mountains with Trimont Ridge, hikers must cross the Little Tennessee River Valley, where Franklin, North Carolina, is located. So bite your lip, tighten your boots, and make the most of it, because after treading nearly 65 miles of the Bartram Trail, the motels, restaurants, grocery stores and laundries of Franklin just might be a good thing. By the way, none of the following route is blazed with any of the yellow Bartram Trail markers.

❀　　❀　　❀

The road walk portion of the Bartram Trail descends past the Buckeye Creek parking area along gravel Buckeye Creek Road. Beyond a few houses, at 0.6 miles, reach Tessentee Creek Road. Turn right here and follow the paved road down Tessentee Creek Valley for 2.2 miles. At mile 2.8, turn right onto Hickory Knoll Road. Stay on Hickory Knoll Road for 2.6 miles. At this point, mile 5.4, Hickory Knoll Road turns right. Continue forward, picking up Clarks Chapel Road. Descend from this intersection, staying on Clarks Chapel Road, for 2.0 miles. At this point, at mile 7.4, turn left on Prentiss Bridge Road, and cross the Little Tennessee River on a road bridge. At mile 7.7, veer right onto Wide Horizon Drive. (This turn is also marked as Bike Route #32.)

Pass a warm-season fruit stand and keep forward for 3.0 miles to reach busy US 441 at mile 10.7. To your right are stores and restaurants. To your right and left are motels, most within a mile's walk. The official Bartram Trail road walk crosses US 441, picking up Belden Road on the other side. Follow Belden Road 0.3 miles, crossing a bridge at mile 11.0. Just past the bridge, turn left onto Roller Mill Road. Climb over a hill, then descend to reach Westgate Plaza on your right at mile 11.8. Here is a grocery store, restaurant, ATM, and laundry. Keep forward to shortly pass under US 64 at mile 12.0, then turn left on Carolina Drive. Follow Carolina Drive 0.2 miles, then turn right on Sloan Road, soon passing the Wayah Ranger Station on your right. Nantahala National Forest information is available here. Just past the ranger station, reach an intersection at mile 12.5. Cross this intersection and pick up Pressley Road. Follow Pressley Road for 1.7 miles to reach the Wallace Branch trailhead and the end of this section and the road walk at mile 14.2. Do not be tempted to turn onto Wallace Branch Road. It does not lead to the Wallace Branch trailhead.

# Bartram Trail, Wallace Branch to Nantahala Lake

| | |
|---|---|
| **Length:** | 18.8 miles |
| **Trail Condition:** | Mostly good |
| **Highs:** | 360-degree vistas from Wayah Bald, rugged ridge walking, solitude between Wine Spring and Nantahala Lake |
| **Lows:** | Limited water and camping, warm-season road access to Wayah Bald |
| **Season:** | Year-round; high country could be rough in winter |
| **Difficulty:** | Strenuous |
| **Use:** | Heavy where BT runs in conjunction with Appalachian Trail, otherwise moderate to low |
| **Tips:** | Plan ahead for water and campsites |
| **Campsites:** | 4, 2.7, 10.2, 12.7 and 18.2 miles |

**WALLACE BRANCH TRAILHEAD:** From the Wayah Ranger Station just north of US 64 and west of downtown Franklin, head north on Sloan Road just a short distance to Old Murphy Road. Cross Old Murphy Road to reach Pressley Road. Keep forward on Pressley Road for 1.7 miles to reach the Wallace Branch trailhead. Do not be tempted to turn left onto Wallace Branch Road. It does not lead to the trailhead. The Bartram Trail starts at the rear of the parking area, immediately spanning a wooden bridge over Wallace Branch.

**NANTAHALA LAKE TRAILHEAD:** From the Wayah Ranger Station just north of US 64 and west of downtown Franklin, head north on Sloan Road just a short distance to Old Murphy Road. Turn left and head west on Old Murphy Road for 3.2 miles to Wayah Road. Turn right on Wayah Road and follow it for 17.9 miles, over Wayah Crest and beside Nantahala Lake to Bateman's Lakeside Store/Phillips 66, on the left. Go inside the store and ask where to park. The parking location is usually near the picnic tables by Wayah Road.

This segment resumes hiking on foot trails through national-forest land. However, end-to-end hikers' relief at having completed the road walk portion of the Bartram Trail may soon turn into disdain: the BT goes up and down, up and down, and ever up along Trimont Ridge, leading to weary legs and shot lungs. Pass by wildlife clearings and a closed, hazardous mica mine before intersecting the Appalachian Trail near Wayah Bald. Climb in conjunction with the AT to reach Wayah Bald and the crest of the Nantahala Mountains. Atop this peak is a stone observation tower with informative signs that will amaze you as much as the view of an endless sea of mountains. The AT and BT continue together another couple of miles to reach Wine Spring, a fine source of water equal to its name. Here, the trails part ways and the Bartram Trail follows a lonely path along McDonald Ridge away from the Nantahalas, making a rugged and spectacular ridge walk to descend precipitously to Nantahala Lake. Cruise along the lake before reaching a store and campground where limited food and supplies can be purchased. The campground has showers and should you want to step to the next level of luxury, cabins. The campground marks the end of this section.

❋    ❋    ❋

Leave the Wallace Branch trailhead and span Wallace Branch on a wooden bridge to enter a forest full of tulip trees on an ascending single-track footpath. Shortly thereafter, look for two waterfalls. The first one flows from a feeder branch above the trail to your right. The second one is on Wallace Branch below to your left. At 0.4 miles, a side trail leads left downhill to a campsite on Wallace Branch. The BT ascends into pine woods, crossing a grassy forest road and a small feeder branch. This is the last water that crosses the trail for 9 miles. Ascend to reach the crest of Trimont Ridge at mile 1.3. To your right, the officially abandoned Trimont Ridge Trail, which is still shown on the latest Nantahala National Forest map, heads east toward Wolfpen Gap. Keep on the BT by turning left, heading west on Trimont Ridge. At mile 1.7, at a sharp right turn in the trail, an unmaintained trail leads left toward Gibson Knob. The BT continues on, circling around Bruce Knob to reach a narrow gap, then ascends. At mile 2.1, look left for short trail leading to a rock shelf and view from William's Pulpit, named after a dedicated Bartram Trail volunteer. Continue over the nose of an unnamed knob, then descend to reach deep Locust Tree Gap at mile 2.7. This is the first of two Locust Tree Gaps on this section. Down the gap to the right are a small campsite on an old roadbed and a small yet reliable spring. You may need to walk down the spring to get a decent flow. This is the last campsite with water for 7 miles.

Climb steeply out of Locust Tree Gap toward Wilkes Knob. Reach a high point at mile 3.4, with the bulk of Wilkes Knob to your right. Begin a descent among large pine, oak, and tulip trees, reaching a gap at mile 3.6. Ascend from this gap, and descend to reach another gap just north of Wildcat Knob at mile 4.1. By now you should begin to see and feel the up-and-down pattern of the trail as it follows Trimont Ridge. Climb steeply, keeping west of Wildcat Knob, picking up a woods road before making Poplar Cove Gap at mile 4.9. Hemlock trees grace the gap, named for a cove on the upper reaches of Mill Creek, located to the southwest. Criss-cross a few small knobs before descending to make Harrison Gap at mile 5.5.

FR 713 enters Harrison Gap from your left and two gated forest roads lie to your right. Bisect the gravel parking area and resume the climb, curving around the north side of a knob, shortly regaining the crest. Continue along the ridge, experiencing more up and down walking among big oak and tulip trees. In spots, the ridge becomes knife-like, with mountain laurel flanking the trail. Descend steeply to reach the second Locust Tree Gap at mile 7.6. Note the atypical grassy forest road cutting through the gap's low point. Keep forward, ascending on the grassy roadbed to soon enter a meadow-like wildlife clearing. Stay on the left side of the clearing, picking up a narrow woods road. At mile 7.8, the Bartram Trail abruptly leaves the woods road and goes right, uphill past a "Hiker Trail" sign. Keep ascending as the trailbed becomes rockier. Follow the switchback upward, breaking the 4,000-foot mark. Regain the crest of Trimont Ridge to reach a second wildlife clearing at mile 8.7. Stay to the left of this clearing and re-enter woods. Birch trees become more common as elevation increases.

Soon, pass through a gap and begin an intense climb. Reach a fenced area on a switchback at mile 9.4. To your left, on the far side of the fence, is an abandoned mica mine. Stay away from here—only fools explore closed mines. Turn uphill away from the mine on an old roadbed. As the trail levels off at mile 9.6, the old roadbed veers left and enters an inholding (private property inside a national forest). The Bartram Trail, however, veers right and descends alongside a steep drop to the right. Do not miss this right turn. Gradually curve to the west and reach a stream at mile 10.1. The stream flowing here is stained brown from tree tannin, but is fine to drink from as long as it's treated. At mile 10.2, the BT intersects the Appalachian Trail. To the right is an overused campsite on a slight slope.

The BT turns left here, now running in conjunction with the AT. The trail tread becomes much more worn. Ascend past an intermittent spring, breaking the 5,000-foot mark. The rocky, rooty trailbed rises to meet a closed road at mile 10.6. Keep climbing past the road. The forest canopy opens overhead before reaching the clearing and tower of Wayah Bald, 5,348 feet, at mile 10.8. This is the highest point of the entire Bartram Trail. The interesting stone tower was built by Civilian Conservation Corps members in the 1930s. The original tower was taller, but was destroyed by a fire. Interpretive signs tell of the bald and tower's history as well as what mountains are on the horizon, from Georgia's Rabun Bald to Tennessee's highest point, Clingmans Dome, in the Smokies.

The BT continues to follow the AT, descending along the paved path leading downhill from the tower. Pass more interpretive information before the trail splits right at mile 10.9, just past some rest rooms for drive-up visitors. Keep just below the ridgecrest and Wayah Road, among specimens of a northern hardwood forest—beech, sugar maple, yellow birch, cherry, and striped maple. Cross a grassy roadbed at an angle at mile 11.1. Keep west, passing nearly pure beech stands on a single-track path. Curve around Rocky Bald Ridge, bisecting several dry washes. At mile 12.5, intersect a woods road and veer right, keeping downhill. (This road leads left to Wine Spring Bald.) Ahead (the road turns to the right), stay forward to reach Wine Spring at mile 12.7. This rocked-in water source lives up to its name, and is good as wine to the thirsty hiker. Campsites are situated near the water source and ahead where the Bartram Trail and Appalachian Trail diverge. Mountain holly is prevalent around this spring.

At the junction, the AT continues forward, while the BT turns right and once again becomes narrow. Begin a pleasant high country forest cruise in a mix of northern hardwoods and oaks. Enter a wildlife clearing at mile 13.0. Keep walking to the very far end of the clearing, avoiding the roadbed leaving the right hand side of the meadow. The yellow-blazed Bartram Trail leaves the meadow as a single-track footpath, running roughly parallel to the Wine Spring Creek drainage. Moderately descend to reach a second wildlife clearing at mile 13.8. This clearing is broken with oak trees. On the left side of the meadow is a "Danger: Rifle Range" sign. The BT leaves the upper right hand side of this meadow, now on an old jeep trail. The walking is easy and glorious. Reach a third wildlife meadow at mile 14.5. Cut straight across the grass and steeply descend through hemlock to reach paved FR 711 and Sawmill Gap at mile 14.7. Pass around the metal forest service gate, then cross the paved road near a vista point and re-enter the woods.

Ascend away from Sawmill Gap, passing around a second metal gate. Climb to regain the ridgecrest. At mile 15.6, look for a faint side trail on an old roadbed leading right; this spur trail leads to some views at the brushy peak of Jarrett Bald. Now comes the tough part. Continuing past the spur trail, the ridgeline narrows. Rock outcrops burst forth from the soil. The BT winds and drops and twists and turns among hemlocks, hardwoods, and rhododendron. Smart hikers will constantly watch their footing. Woe to those coming up the other direction from Nantahala Lake. At mile 17.0, the trail makes a conspicuous left turn, then descends to meet a trail junction at mile 17.3. Here, a faint trail with large green blazes painted on trees goes left. Keep descending. The drops get steeper, even with switchbacks that pass beneath deep, dark hemlock copses. Come alongside a streamlet before reaching Wayah Road at mile 18.1. Turn right on the two-lane paved highway. Wine Spring Creek flows into Nantahala Lake under the highway by culvert. Backpackers can consider taking the unmaintained trail up Wine Spring Creek away from Wayah Road into National Forest land for a campsite with water.

Circle around Nantahala Lake on Wayah Road, passing Lake's End Restaurant, which has food and a phone. Reach Bateman's Lakeside Camp Store and the end of this section at mile 18.8. The store has limited food and supplies, a campground with showers, and cabins. From here, the BT turns left away from Wayah Road just past the "Phillips 66" sign.

# Bartram Trail, Nantahala Lake to Winding Stairs

| | |
|---|---|
| **Length:** | 17.3 miles |
| **Trail Condition:** | Mostly good |
| **Highs:** | Piercy Creek valley, views from Rattlesnake Knob area |
| **Lows:** | Gravel road walk below Nantahala Dam |
| **Season:** | Year-round; best during spring, early summer and fall |
| **Difficulty:** | Moderate to difficult |
| **Use:** | Low to moderate |
| **Tips:** | Beginning portion through a mix of public and private land is challenging to follow, stay with yellow blazes |
| **Campsites:** | 1.8, 2.3, 5.9, 8.3, and 10.5 miles |

**NANTAHALA LAKE TRAILHEAD:** From the Wayah Ranger Station just north of US 64 and west of downtown Franklin, head north on Sloan Road just a short distance to Old Murphy Road. Turn left and head west on Old Murphy Road for 3.2 miles to Wayah Road. Turn right on Wayah Road and follow it for 17.9 miles, over Wayah Crest and beside Nantahala Lake to Bateman's Lakeside Store/Phillips 66. Go inside the store and ask where to park. The parking area is usually near the picnic tables by Wayah Road.

**WINDING STAIRS TRAILHEAD:** From Andrews, North Carolina, take US 19/US 129 north for a little over 6 miles to the point where US 129 turns left. At this point, keep forward on US 19 for 3.6 miles to the Winding Stairs parking area, on your right. This parking area is hard to see until you are right on it. Look for white pedestrian crossing markers crossing US 19 at the right turn into the Winding Stairs parking area. A Bartram Trail information sign is located in the parking area.

This section of the Bartram Trail roughly follows the Nantahala River downstream from Nantahala Lake toward the Nantahala Gorge made famous by rafters, canoeists, and kayakers. "Roughly follows" is a good description for two reasons: the trail is hard to follow in places because it repeatedly jumps on and off old logging roads at its beginning, and despite the perceived level nature of the riverside, it makes a lot of ups and downs along the entire section.

Begin by leaving the Lakeside Store and pass through a jumble of confusing roads and foot trails as the path skirts around Nantahala Lake and behind Nantahala Dam on and off private property. Cross the Nantahala River on a concrete ford that is less scary than it sounds, then join a quiet gravel road for a couple of miles along the river to reach National Forest land near Appletree Group Camp. The trail passes through attractive riverside woods here, going up and down like a roller coaster, before turning away from the river at Poplar Cove Creek and heading toward beautiful Piercy Creek. Head up this attractive valley, then swing around Rattlesnake Knob with many views through the trees. From a high point, make a continuous descent to reach the Nantahala River near the boat launch site and pick up a paved trail that runs along the river to end at Winding Stairs parking area. Campsites and water are plentiful, even with the mix of private and public land.

❀    ❀    ❀

The Bartram Trail leaves the Lakeside Store, heading north, away from Nantahala Lake. At the end of the store parking lot is a "Phillips 66" sign. Turn left here, down an unlikely gravel road that passes just below a house to your right. The road spans Lee Branch by culvert, then curves right. Watch carefully at mile 0.2, as the BT turns acutely left onto a logging road grown up with young trees. Curve back toward Nantahala Lake, ascending among tulip trees and white pines. Cross a spring branch at 0.5 miles. The trail then picks up a gravel road leading left toward a house. Follow this road just a short distance, then veer right onto an older road. Walk the older road just a short distance, then turn left onto a single-track footpath. Take this single-track footpath as it switchbacks to the right and hits yet another gravel road at 0.8 miles. Turn left on this gravel road, following it 0.1 miles. On a left curve the BT leaves the gravel road right, paralleling the road from above. Ascend, picking up a view of Nantahala Dam through the trees as the trail curves around the lake. At mile 1.7, turn left off the single-track and pick up a woods road heading down a streamlet on your right. Ahead, at mile 1.8, is a campsite near rhododendron where the BT crosses the small stream. The BT punches through the rhododendron thickets to meet an old road coming in on your right at mile 2.2, then begins to descend toward the river. Watch carefully as the trail abruptly turns left to enter a neat campsite overlooking a waterfall. Be apprised that although you can see the waterfall, accessing water in the ultra steep terrain is another matter.

The BT returns to the road it was on, then switchbacks down to reach Nantahala Dam Road after some steps at mile 2.7. Stay left here and cross the concrete ford of the clear Nantahala River. At this point, the Nantahala has been emasculated, with much of its flow diverted from the riverbed and sent by penstock, a pipe regulating water flow, from the lake several miles to a power station near the end of this section. Near the power station, the Bartram Trail actually heads over the piped water by bridge just before it re-enters the river.

Ascend from the river ford and turn right onto Highwater Trail Road, a gravel road with a few houses on it. Continue down the quiet road. You may hear cars at mile 3.7—paved Junaluska Road lies on the other side of the river. A piped spring emerges from rock to your left past the point where Highwater Trail Road nears Junaluska Road. At mile 4.7, intersect gravel Cloudwalker Cove Road and turn right, passing under the penstock. Soon, reach paved Junaluska Road and turn right. Walk down the road a bit to reach the entrance to Appletree Group Camp at mile 4.9. Head straight for the entrance sign, then step over the split-rail fence. The Bartram Trail once again travels alongside the river, now beneath a long tunnel of rhododendron.

At mile 5.1, the BT veers left and joins an old forest road that passes alongside a pretty field that is part of the group camp. Ahead is a picnic area with covered picnic shelters. At mile 5.3, just after nearing a group campsite, the BT passes around a metal gate and heads up a closed forest road. At mile 5.4, the BT abruptly turns right, downhill, as a single-track footpath. Drop down to the Nantahala River and a campsite situated among the pines and hemlocks. This is one of the most attractive sections of the BT. Campers be apprised that moderately-used, gravel Old River Road is across the water. At mile 5.9, reach a campsite beneath tulip trees on an elevated flat. Curve left with the Nantahala, then ascend, picking up an obvious roadbed to step over Walnut Cove Creek at mile 7.0. Head upstream in a narrow cove, then switchback toward the Nantahala, passing through an open tulip tree woodland. Descend a V-shaped hollow to step over Poplar Cove Creek at mile 7.5. Pick up a roadbed, descending back to the Nantahala before climbing steeply from the river.

Follow switchbacks leading south, passing a white pine plantation, before crossing Poplar Cove Creek by culvert at mile 8.2. The cove here is choked in rhododendron, but ahead, to the right of the trail, is a little-used campsite in a hardwood-hemlock flat. Other small campsites lie among the rhododendron. Keep ascending the cove in rhododendron, passing the remnants of a bridge over a side stream. The rhododendron gives way to hardwoods as the BT circles around the upper end of the cove, passing left through a gap at mile 8.9. Keep ascending, passing Turkey Pen Cove down to your right. The Nantahala River is clearly audible far below, and the Nantahala Mountains are visible across the river valley. Pass through a second gap before entering a wildlife clearing at mile 9.3. Stay on the upper end of the clearing, taking a timber road from the clearing. Just past the clearing is a confusing intersection of old timber roads. The BT takes a faint single-track path to the right, then picks up a timber road, which then turns left. Stay with the yellow blazes.

Make a pleasant descent on the timber road. At mile 10.1, the BT passes through a gap and enters a white pine plantation. Needles carpet the trailway. Drop down to Piercy Creek, reaching a feeder stream just before crossing Piercy Creek itself. This crossing can be dry footed at normal flow. Turn left, heading up Piercy Creek beneath towering white pines, and reach a trail junction at mile 10.5. Here, the blue-blazed Piercy Creek Trail heads downstream to reach the Nantahala River and a major ford. A side trail leads left to one of several campsites in the vicinity.

Keep forward on the BT, stepping over a small tributary and enter a wind-damaged forest. At mile 10.7, in the middle of the fallen trees, lies a trail junction. The Laurel Creek Trail leaves left toward Appletree Group Camp. Continue forward, picking up an old road that makes a steady ascent beneath laurel tunnels. At mile 11.3, the trail nears Laurel

Branch on your left before switchbacking right to climb in attractive pine-laurel-oak forest. Reach another trail junction at mile 11.7. The London Bald Trail keeps forward on the old roadbed while the Bartram Trail turns acutely right as a single-track path.

Keep ascending, winding into hollows and out along rib ridges. The thinly forested rib ridges offer vistas to the north and east as the trailbed becomes more rocky. At mile 13.1, at a double blaze, the trail turns sharply left and picks up a narrow woods road. Shortly cut through a little gap. The hulking bulk of Cheoah Bald, the Bartram Trail terminus, becomes visible to your right. Descend in light rhododendron, leaving the roadbed to cross a small branch at mile 13.4. Just above the path, a low-flow waterfall issues over a rockface. Ahead, descend by many switchbacks on a piney slope into the Nantahala Gorge. The houses of Topton and the Snowbird Mountains to the west are visible. At mile 14.1, pass by a light-green water surge tank and keep descending, now on a wide gravel access road. Blazes are infrequent on this road. At mile 14.9, a road comes in on your right—keep forward and reach a road fork—keep right, downhill. The tree canopy gives way as the BT nears a power station. Watch for the trail turning left off the access road at mile 15.8. Descend through a brushy area and pass a Bartram Trail signboard. Keep downhill, reaching Wayah Road below.

Turn right on Wayah Road, keeping the power station to your right. Bridge the outflow of water from the power station, the same water that traveled through the penstock, then immediately turn left, stepping over a guardrail at mile 16.0. This is a busy area where paddlers enter the river. Join the paved bike trail that spans the Nantahala on an iron bridge.

The BT traces the bike trail through bottomland wooded in sycamore and tulip trees. At mile 16.3, look left as the river splits around an island. Paddlers will be visible here. Continue along the Nantahala, as the bike path comes very close to the river near a wood fence. At the end of this fence, at mile 17.2, turn left onto Winding Stairs Road and bridge the Nantahala as it works around both sides of another island. Just past this bridge, reach the Winding Stairs parking area and the end of this section. From here, the BT keeps forward, crossing US 19, and heads for its terminus at Cheoah Bald.

# Bartram Trail, Winding Stairs to Cheoah Bald

| | |
|---|---|
| **Length:** | 5.1 miles |
| **Trail Condition:** | Good |
| **Highs:** | View from Cheoah Bald, northern terminus of Bartram Trail, waterfalls of Ledbetter Creek |
| **Lows:** | Steepest section of entire trail |
| **Season:** | Year-round, Cheoah Bald could be very cold in winter |
| **Difficulty:** | Strenuous |
| **Use:** | Moderate, heavy on Cheoah Bald where Appalachian Trail passes by |
| **Tips:** | No auto access from the top of Cheoah Bald; you must either backtrack to Winding Stairs or take AT 4.4 miles to Stecoah Gap near Robbinsville or 7.8 miles to Wesser in Nantahala Gorge |
| **Campsites:** | 0.4, 2.1, and 3.9 miles |

**WINDING STAIRS TRAILHEAD:** From Andrews, North Carolina, take US 19/US 129 north for a little over 6 miles to the point where US 129 turns left. At this point, keep forward on US 19 for 3.6 more miles to the Winding Stairs parking area, on your right. This parking area is hard to see until you are right on it. Look for white pedestrian crossing markers crossing US 19 at the right turn into the Winding Stairs parking area. A Bartram Trail information sign is located in the gravel parking area.

**CHEOAH BALD TRAILHEAD:** Cheoah Bald is accessible only by foot. If you choose to exit Cheoah Bald using the Appalachian Trail, Wesser is north of Winding Stairs parking area on US 19. Parking is available at Nantahala Outdoor Center, across the river from US 19. Ask someone from NOC exactly where to park if you are going for several days. Stecoah Gap parking area is east of Robbinsville on NC 143. The AT crosses NC 143 at Stecoah Gap. Parking is available at the gap.

This section is the grand finale of the Bartram Trail, and it lives up to expectations of what a long-trail grand finale should be. The BT climbs out of the Nantahala Gorge into the steep and narrow Ledbetter Creek valley. The valley is cloaked in a northern hardwood forest, shading waterfall after waterfall. Ledbetter Creek eventually runs out of water as the Bartram Trail reaches the high country to meet the Appalachian Trail for a final short section to reach Cheoah Bald. The vistas here are fantastic. From a mountain meadow, you can look to the east and south, to the mountains over which the Bartram Trail passed. And from a rugged rock outcrop, you can look to the rampart of the Great Smoky Mountains, looming in the west. Both sunrise and sunset here can be memorable, but this beauty comes with a price. This is easily the steepest section of the BT, and the climb is nearly continuous from the bottom of the Nantahala Gorge to the top of the bald. And once you reach the bald, you can't just stroll to the car. You have three options, one of which you will want to choose before you reach to the top of the mountain: A) Backtrack to Winding Stairs parking area; B) Hike the Appalachian Trail north to Stecoah Gap and NC 143; or C) Hike the Appalachian Trail south to Wesser in the lower Nantahala Gorge. Backtracking doesn't require two cars or a shuttle; the hike to Stecoah Gap is the shortest way out from Cheoah Bald, and the hike to Wesser has the easiest shuttle but is the longest by foot. You make the call. After the climb, you will understand why the Cherokee word Nantahala means "land of the noonday sun."

Campsites with water are located at fairly even intervals along the trail—0.4, 2.1, and 3.9 miles. I do not recommend camping at the bald, as the campsites are worn and need a rest. Also, no water is available on the bald. Sassafras Gap trail shelter is located on the AT a mile east from Cheoah Bald toward Wesser.

❊     ❊     ❊

Start this section by leaving Winding Stairs parking area and walking across US 19. Be careful here, as the road is fairly busy, especially on warm weekends, when the whole gorge is hopping. Keep forward, crossing the tracks of the Great Smoky Mountain Railroad. Ascend under a power line through a brushy area, re-entering the woods. Turn left, upstream in the Nantahala Gorge, then descend by switchbacks to reach

Ledbetter Creek at 0.4 miles. Cross an unmaintained trail heading up the creek just before reaching Ledbetter Creek and a campsite. Rock-hop Ledbetter Creek. This is the first of several creek crossings, all of which can be dry-footed in times of normal flow.

At this point, begin the ascent from the Nantahala Gorge, angling up the mountainside in a rich forest. Make some wide switchbacks as the forest evolves from deciduous trees to more pines. These open piney areas avail views across the gorge. The surge tank the BT passed by is plainly visible across the river. Reach a gap at mile 1.2. Pick up an old roadbed and keep ascending through brush and young trees. Reach a more substantial old road at mile 1.4 and keep right. Just ahead is an unmaintained side trail leading left through mountain laurel toward Handpole Branch. Make a steady descent with broken views through the trees and tunnels of rhododendron, reaching Ledbetter Creek at mile 1.8. Rock-hop the watercourse just above a long pool, into which falls a wide, two-tiered cascade. Circle around a cove, now in a forest of northern hardwoods such as yellow birch and beech. Step over a side branch of Ledbetter Creek where parts of an old stove remain, probably from a former hunting camp. Just past the side branch, reach a camping flat beside Ledbetter Creek at mile 2.1. This is the widest area of the whole creek valley.

Ascend away from the flat and rock-hop to the left bank of Ledbetter Creek at mile 2.3. Pick up a faint roadbed, passing burned forest to your left. The fire didn't make it into this moist and narrow valley, but stayed on the drier, more exposed ridgeline. The valley narrows and steepens. Blankets of rhododendron add to the crowded sense of the area. Leave the faint roadbed. This is where the serious climbing resumes. Take time to look at the rugged bluffline across the crashing stream. Tiny feeder branches and seeps enter the valley. At mile 2.8, as the trail curves right, pass Bartram Falls, a series of tiered drops. Ahead, the stream slices a slender course in a vertical rock chute. At mile 3.0, cross Ledbetter Creek atop the series of waterfalls. You are now on the right-hand side of the creek. Keep uphill, picking your way through a rock jumble just before stepping over a side stream, over which bridge beams are still visible.

The valley narrows again. Step over Ledbetter Creek at mile 3.2, and at mile 3.3. You are once again on the right-hand side of the creek. Climb

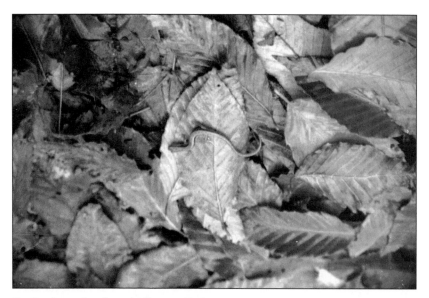

Small salamander along the Bartram Trail

through a forest of beech and birch broken by spring seeps cloaked in rhododendron. The creek is now a good distance away. Meet a seemingly improbable old road coming around the mountain at mile 3.8. Trace the grade as it keeps forward to meet Ledbetter Creek again at mile 3.9. Step over the watercourse, which can nearly dry up in fall, though a spring is very near on the far side of the drainage. The tiny flat has been used as a campsite in the past. Keep ascending beyond the flat to meet grassy FR 259 at mile 4.1. Also known as Nolton Ridge Road, this vehicle access road is open only in the month of October, though it is gated year-round a half mile to your left. This section of the road is used by forest service personnel to maintain the meadow on Cheoah Bald. FR 259 is accessed from Ledbetter Road, off US 129.

Start the third super-steep climb of this section. The on-and-off stream to your right is the last water from here to Cheoah Bald. Circle around the head of a cove to mercifully level off and make Bellcollar Gap at mile 4.7. Keep right here, ascending by switchbacks to meet the Appalachian Trail at mile 4.9. Turn right on the AT, heading toward Cheoah Bald. Make the final ascent on a knife-edge ridge among stunted trees and low rhododendron, running in conjunction with the AT. Break out onto the perimeter of a large meadow to your right. The views open with it. Keep forward to reach the high point of Cheoah Bald, 5,062 feet, and the end of the Bartram Trail at mile 5.1. A sign indicates Cheoah Bald, and a blue-blazed side trail leads left to a rock outcrop and a panoramic view of the Great Smoky Mountains on the horizon. Here, hikers must decide how to descend the summit of Cheoah Bald, by either backtracking on the BT, or taking the AT to either Wesser or Stecoah Gap. You might want to contemplate your decision for a while. After all, that climb from the gorge was a humdinger.

## Bartram Trail Log

### RUSSELL BRIDGE TO WARWOMAN DELL

| | | |
|---|---|---|
| 0.0 | 110.7 | Bartram Trail leaves GA 28 parking area |
| 0.1 | 110.6 | Intersect woods road, cross West Fork Chattooga on metal bridge |
| 1.2 | 109.5 | Span Holden Creek on footbridge |
| 2.2 | 108.5 | Leave flat with homesite near pine copse |
| 2.5 | 108.2 | Intersect horse trail |
| 3.2 | 107.5 | Span Bynum Branch on footbridge, campsite |
| 4.1 | 106.6 | Cross Laurel Branch in rhododendron |
| 4.3 | 106.4 | Cross unnamed stream, sloped campsite |
| 5.9 | 104.8 | Intersect wide, road-like horse trail |
| 6.1 | 104.6 | Faint side trail leads right to campsite on Warwoman Creek |
| 6.3 | 104.4 | Span Warwoman Creek on metal footbridge |
| 6.5 | 104.2 | Cross gravel Earls Ford, beaten up campsites |
| 7.8 | 102.9 | Reach flat on Chattooga River, campsites |
| 8.3 | 102.4 | Leave Chattooga River for good |
| 9.1 | 101.6 | Side trail leads left to top end of Dicks Creek Falls, soon cross Dicks Creek on ridge, campsites in area |
| 9.5 | 101.2 | Reach Sandy Ford Road, begin ascending ridge |
| 11.0 | 99.7 | Span dry streambed on footbridge |
| 11.4 | 99.3 | Reach Speed Gap, ascend |
| 12.9 | 97.8 | Reach Bob Gap, cross gravel Pool Ridge Road |
| 13.3 | 97.4 | BT picks up woods road, climb over knobs |
| 14.7 | 96.0 | Leave old roadbed on sharp right turn |
| 14.9 | 95.8 | Small campsite |
| 15.1 | 95.6 | Pass small stream in rhododendron thicket |
| 15.9 | 94.8 | Reach crest of Rainy Ridge, keep forward |

## Bartram Trail Log *(continued)*

| | | |
|---|---|---|
| **16.1** | **94.6** | Unexpected right turn off old woods road |
| **17.0** | **93.7** | "Goat Trail" intersects from left, BT descends forward with "Goat Trail" |
| **17.3** | **93.4** | Reach Green Gap, "Goat Trail" leaves left, BT ascends |
| **17.7** | **93.0** | Southward view of Lake Toccoa |
| **18.6** | **92.1** | Reach Warwoman Dell Picnic Area, trailside parking, water spigot in warm season |

### WARWOMAN DELL TO HALE RIDGE ROAD

| | | |
|---|---|---|
| **18.8** | **91.9** | Cross paved Warwoman Road, ascend past Becky Falls and enter burned area |
| **19.1** | **91.6** | Pass bulldozed firebreak |
| **19.6** | **91.1** | Span streamlet on footbridge |
| **20.6** | **90.1** | Reach camping flat along Martin Creek |
| **20.7** | **90.0** | Side trail leads right past rock house and to base of Martin Creek Falls |
| **22.1** | **88.6** | Side trail leads left to top of Pinnacle Knob |
| **22.4** | **88.3** | Courthouse Gap, ascend around east side of Hogback |
| **23.6** | **87.1** | Step over tiny streamlet, campsite on roadbed up and to left of water |
| **23.9** | **86.8** | Gap north of Raven Knob, dry campsite, ascend Rock Mountain |
| **24.8** | **85.9** | Pick up old road, swing around northwest side of Rock Mountain |
| **25.7** | **85.0** | Windy Gap |
| **26.6** | **84.1** | Step over pair of small streams |
| **27.1** | **83.6** | Reach Wilson Gap, keep forward on FR 155 |
| **27.6** | **83.1** | Bartram Trail leaves left from FR 155, slabbing around Double Knob |
| **28.8** | **81.9** | Reach Gap between Wilson Knob and Flat Top, dry campsite |
| **29.1** | **81.6** | Side trail leads left to view from rockface |
| **29.2** | **81.5** | Spring branch and campsite on left in thicket, enter prescribed burn area, views |
| **30.2** | **80.5** | Saltrock Gap, campsite |
| **30.4** | **80.3** | BT leaves right, water accessible on trail leading forward |
| **30.9** | **79.8** | Tiny spring crosses trail |
| **31.3** | **79.4** | Flint Gap, side trail leaves left for Flint Knob, BT ascends by switchbacks |
| **32.1** | **78.6** | Reach top of Rabun Bald, wooden platform at stone tower offers 360-degree views. Three Forks Trail leaves right for Hale Ridge Road, BT descends |

## Bartram Trail Log *(continued)*

### HALE RIDGE ROAD TO BUCKEYE CREEK

| | | |
|---|---|---|
| **32.8** | **77.9** | Rough road leads left to Beegum Gap, BT keeps right |
| **33.7** | **77.0** | Bisect gravel road leading left to nearby house |
| **34.2** | **76.5** | Span clear stream on two wooden bridges connected by small island, many small bridges ahead |
| **35.1** | **75.6** | Span stream on bridge, cross overgrown road, sloped campsite downhill to right |
| **35.8** | **74.9** | Bridge stream below low-volume waterfall spilling over rockface |
| **36.1** | **74.6** | Campsite on right after bridge over small stream, Hale Ridge Road very near |
| **36.2** | **74.5** | Reach Hale Ridge Road, descend along road Hale Ridge Road to Buckeye Creek |

### BUCKEYE CREEK TO WALLACE BRANCH

| | | |
|---|---|---|
| **36.3** | **74.4** | Enter woods on left and soon reach North Carolina and Nantahala National Forest |
| **37.2** | **73.5** | Curve left at gap on Osage Mountain |
| **37.8** | **72.9** | Campsite on roadbed downhill to right after spring seep |
| **38.9** | **71.8** | Intersect Hurrah Ridge Trail, BT stays left |
| **39.3** | **71.4** | Intersect West Fork Trail, small campsite, BT ascends toward NC 106 |
| **39.5** | **71.2** | Intersect blue-blazed side trail looping toward NC 106, keep left |
| **39.9** | **70.8** | Reach paved NC 106, cross road and ascend |
| **40.2** | **70.5** | Side trail leads left to waterfall, BT crosses stream above fall, ascend Scaly Mountain by switchbacks |
| **40.8** | **69.9** | Turn sharply right on roadbed, views to the south |
| **41.3** | **69.4** | Access trail leads right down to Hickory Knut Road, BT veers sharply left |
| **41.8** | **68.9** | Top of Scaly Mountain, 4,804 feet, views aplenty |
| **42.2** | **68.5** | Reach Gall Tree Gap after descending, keep descending among rhododendron |
| **42.9** | **67.8** | Descent moderates between sections of switchbacks |
| **44.3** | **66.4** | Reach Tessentee Creek, water and campsite, pick up wide roadbed leading right |
| **44.6** | **66.1** | BT leaves roadbed as single-track trail |
| **46.0** | **64.7** | Intersect dirt road, turn right, briefly walk road, then turn left, resuming single-track trail to soon reach crest of Fishhawk Mountains and ascend |
| **46.6** | **64.1** | Side trail leads left to view of Peggy Knob, climb over Keith Day Knob then descend through wildlife clearing |
| **47.1** | **63.6** | Reach Jones Gap and FR 4522, keep forward on grassy lane |

## Bartram Trail Log *(continued)*

| | | |
|---|---|---|
| **47.4** | **63.3** | Intersect blue-blazed spur trail leading left after passing through wildlife clearing, spur trail ascends to top of Jones Knob with great views |
| **48.2** | **62.5** | Reach ridgecrest after swinging around side of Jones Knob, spur trail ahead leads left to views of Whiterock Mountain |
| **48.4** | **62.3** | Whiterock Gap, campsite, spur trail leads right 800 feet to water at Stevens Creek |
| **48.8** | **61.9** | Spur trail leads right short distance to small spring |
| **48.9** | **61.8** | Blue-blazed spur trail leads left to top of Whiterock Mountain, great views, Bartram Trail leads right to Little Fishhawk Mountain |
| **49.4** | **61.3** | Reach high point on Little Fishhawk Mountain, descend to gap |
| **49.9** | **60.8** | Blue-blazed spur trail leads right, to top of Fishhawk Mountain where plaque commemorates William Bartram, BT swings around west side of Fishhawk Mountain. |
| **50.8** | **59.9** | Reach small gap between Fishhawk Mountain and Wolf Rock |
| **51.3** | **59.4** | Great views from Wolf Rock Overlook |
| **51.9** | **58.8** | Bisect gap where old road crosses ridgeline |
| **52.6** | **58.1** | Pass by dilapidated school bus that was part of old hunting camp |
| **53.0** | **57.7** | BT leaves ridgeline left at gap, dry campsite, descend toward Buckeye Creek |
| **53.8** | **56.9** | Reach roadbed at intermittent stream |
| **54.0** | **56.7** | Reach second roadbed, turn right |
| **54.2** | **56.5** | Stream flows under roadbed via culvert, keep descending |
| **55.0** | **55.7** | Span tiny creek by culvert |
| **55.3** | **55.4** | Pass around forest service gate, soon reach trailside parking with Bartram Trail information on left, begin 14-mile road walk through Franklin and Little Tennessee River Valley on Buckeye Creek Road |

### WALLACE BRANCH TO NANTAHALA LAKE

| | | |
|---|---|---|
| **55.9** | **54.8** | Turn right on Tessentee Creek Road |
| **58.1** | **52.6** | Turn right on Hickory Knoll Road |
| **60.7** | **50.0** | Stay forward, picking up Clarks Chapel Road |
| **62.7** | **48.0** | Turn left on Prentiss Bridge Road, span Little Tennessee River |
| **63.0** | **47.7** | Turn right onto Wide Horizon Drive |
| **66.0** | **44.7** | Reach US 441, restaurants, stores, motels within 1 mile both left and right, official Bartram Trail crosses 441 and keeps forward on Belden Road |
| **66.3** | **44.4** | After crossing creek on bridge, turn left onto Roller Mill Road, climb hill |
| **67.1** | **43.6** | Westgate Plaza on right, grocery store, laundry, restaurant, and 24-hour ATM |

## Bartram Trail Log *(continued)*

| | | |
|---|---|---|
| **67.3** | **43.4** | Pass under US 64, then turn left on Carolina Drive |
| **67.5** | **43.2** | Turn right on Sloan Road, soon passing Wayah Ranger Station |
| **67.8** | **42.9** | Intersect Old Murphy Road, keep forward, picking up Pressley Road, stay forward on Pressley Road, ignoring left turn on Wallace Branch Road |
| **69.5** | **41.2** | Reach Wallace Branch trailhead, trailside parking, BT crosses Wallace Branch on wooden footbridge, yellow blazes resume |
| **69.9** | **40.8** | After passing waterfall on feeder stream, reach side trail leading left to campsite on Buckeye Creek, shortly step over feeder branch after grassy forest road, last water crossing BT for 9 miles |
| **70.8** | **39.9** | Reach crest of Trimont Ridge, BT turns left along ridgeline |
| **71.2** | **39.5** | Unmaintained trail leads left toward Gibson Knob |
| **71.6** | **39.1** | Spur trail leads left to rock shelf and view from Williams Pulpit |
| **72.2** | **38.5** | Locust Tree Gap, campsite on roadbed and small spring downhill to right |
| **72.9** | **37.8** | Reach high point on side of Wilkes Knob |
| **73.6** | **37.1** | Gap just north of Wilkes Knob |
| **74.4** | **36.3** | Reach Poplar Cove Gap, criss-cross a few small knobs |
| **75.0** | **35.7** | Harrison Gap, FR 713 enters from left, BT keeps forward straight up hill |
| **77.1** | **33.6** | Reach second Locust Tree Gap in this section, ascend grassy forest road to wildlife clearing |
| **77.3** | **33.4** | BT leaves right from woods road, up toward "Hiker Trail" sign |
| **78.2** | **32.5** | Pass through wildlife clearing |
| **78.9** | **31.8** | Abandoned mica mine on far side of fence at switchback, keep uphill on old road |
| **79.1** | **31.6** | BT keeps right, old road turns left toward private inholding |
| **79.6** | **31.1** | Reach stream after descending |
| **79.7** | **31.0** | Intersect AT, campsite to right, BT and AT head uphill toward Wayah Bald |
| **80.1** | **30.6** | Bisect closed grassy road |
| **80.3** | **30.4** | Reach stone tower atop Wayah Bald, 360-degree views |
| **80.4** | **30.3** | Leave Wayah Bald area near rest rooms |
| **80.6** | **30.1** | Cross grassy roadbed at an angle, curve around Rocky Bald Ridge |
| **82.0** | **28.7** | Pick up grassy road leading left to Wine Spring Bald, Bartram Trail keeps right down grassy road |
| **82.2** | **28.5** | Reach Wine Spring, campsites in area, Bartram Trail and Appalachian Trail split just ahead, BT leaves right along McDonald Ridge |
| **82.5** | **28.2** | Enter wildlife clearing |

## Bartram Trail Log *(continued)*

| | | |
|---|---|---|
| **83.3** | **27.4** | Reach second wildlife clearing broken with oak trees |
| **84.0** | **26.7** | Reach third wildlife clearing, descend |
| **84.2** | **26.5** | Sawmill Gap, paved FR 711 passes through gap, BT ascends forward |
| **85.1** | **25.6** | Faint side trail leads right on old roadbed to views from Jarrett Bald |
| **86.5** | **24.2** | BT makes conspicuous left turn, descends |
| **86.8** | **23.9** | Faint trail with large green blazes leads left, keep descending |
| **87.6** | **23.1** | Reach Wayah Road after very sharp descent, turn right onto Wayah Road, passing unmaintained trail leading up Wine Spring Creek, campsites |
| **88.4** | **22.3** | Reach Bateman's Lakeside Store after passing Lake's End Restaurant, campground with showers, cabins, and limited items at small camp store |

## NANTAHALA LAKE TO WINDING STAIRS

| | | |
|---|---|---|
| **88.5** | **22.2** | Span Lee Branch via culvert after leaving Wayah Road at "Phillips 66" sign |
| **88.6** | **22.1** | BT turns acutely left, passing small stream, switch between single-track and old roads |
| **90.1** | **20.6** | Trail turns left, descending on woods road beside stream, campsite 0.1 miles ahead |
| **90.6** | **20.1** | Campsite beside waterfall |
| **91.1** | **19.6** | Reach Nantahala Dam Road, turn left, and cross Nantahala on concrete ford, turn right after ford on gravel High Water Trail Road |
| **92.1** | **18.6** | Paved Junaluska Road lies across Nantahala River, piped spring on left |
| **93.1** | **17.6** | BT turns right on Cloudwalker Cove Road |
| **93.3** | **17.4** | Reach Appletree Group Camp, descend along Nantahala River |
| **93.5** | **17.2** | Join roadbed, passing field framed in split-rail fence |
| **93.8** | **16.9** | BT veers right off roadbed after passing around metal gate, campsite beside Nantahala River among pines and hemlocks |
| **94.3** | **16.4** | Campsite on raised flat beneath tulip trees |
| **95.4** | **15.3** | Step over Walnut Cove Creek |
| **95.9** | **14.8** | Step over Poplar Cove Creek, pick up old roadbed and ascend from gorge |
| **96.6** | **14.1** | Span Poplar Cove Creek by culvert, campsite ahead on right |
| **97.3** | **13.4** | Turn left while passing through gap |
| **97.7** | **13.0** | Pass through second gap and enter wildlife clearing |

## Bartram Trail Log *(continued)*

| | | |
|---|---|---|
| **98.5** | **12.2** | Pass through third gap and enter white pine plantation, descend |
| **98.9** | **11.8** | Reach trail junction after crossing Piercy Creek, Piercy Creek Trail leaves right, Bartram Trail keeps forward, campsite to left |
| **99.1** | **11.6** | Trail junction among fallen trees, Laurel Creek Trail leaves left toward Appletree Group Camp, BT keeps forward, now on old road and ascends |
| **100.1** | **10.6** | Reach trail junction, London Bald Trail keeps forward on roadbed, BT turns acutely right on single-track path |
| **101.5** | **9.2** | BT makes sharp left turn at double blaze and picks up narrow woods road |
| **101.8** | **8.9** | Step over small branch above low-flow waterfall, soon descend by switchbacks |
| **102.5** | **8.2** | Pass by light-green water surge tank, descend along access road |
| **103.3** | **7.4** | Keep right as road splits ahead |
| **104.2** | **6.5** | Bartram Trail leaves left off access road, keep downhill and soon reach Wayah Road, turn right on road, keeping power station to your right |
| **104.4** | **6.3** | Bridge outflow coming from power station and turn left after bridge, picking up paved bike trail heading down along Nantahala River |
| **104.7** | **6.0** | Nantahala River splits around an island |
| **105.6** | **5.1** | Leave bike trail and bridge Nantahala River on Winding Stairs Road to reach Winding Stairs trailhead, trailside parking, BT keeps forward to cross US 19 |

### WINDING STAIRS TO CHEOAH BALD

| | | |
|---|---|---|
| **106.0** | **4.7** | Follow trail across brush into woods and reach Ledbetter Creek and campsite |
| **106.8** | **3.9** | Reach gap after ascending from gorge, surge tank is visible across gorge |
| **107.4** | **3.3** | Rock-hop Ledbetter Creek and enter small cove |
| **107.7** | **3.0** | Campsite on left beside Ledbetter Creek |
| **107.9** | **2.8** | Rock-hop Ledbetter Creek, ascend past burned forest to left |
| **108.4** | **2.3** | Bartram Falls on right, many cascades along creek |
| **108.6** | **2.1** | Step over Ledbetter Creek, two more crossings in next 0.3 miles |
| **109.4** | **1.3** | Meet old road coming around the mountainside |
| **109.5** | **1.2** | Cross Ledbetter Creek, old bridge remnants, campsite just beyond crossing |
| **109.7** | **1.0** | Reach grassy and closed FR 259, begin very steep climb |
| **110.3** | **0.4** | Bellcollar Gap, keep ascending |

## Bartram Trail Log *(continued)*

**110.5   0.2**   Intersect Appalachian Trail, turn right, up knife-edge ridge onto perimeter of meadow on Cheoah Bald, views to right

**110.7   0.0**   Reach top of Cheoah Bald, 5,062 feet, and the end of Bartram Trail, blue-blazed spur trail leads left to outcrop and view of Smoky Mountains

## Bartram Trail Information

Chattahoochee National Forest
Tallulah Ranger District
809 Highway 441 South
Clayton, Georgia 30525
www.fs.fed.us/conf

North Carolina Bartram Trail Society
P.O. Box 144
Scaly Mountain, North Carolina
    28775
(828) 526-4904
www.ncbartramtrail.org

Bartram Trail Conference
390 St. Mark's Drive
Lilburn, Georgia 30047
www.bartramtrail.org

Nantahala National Forest
P.O. Box 2750
160A Zillicoa Street
Asheville, North Carolina 28802
(828) 257-4200
www.cs.unca.edu/nfsnc

Nantahala National Forest
Highlands Ranger District
2010 Flat Mountain Road
Highlands, North Carolina
(828) 526-3765

Nantahala National Forest
Wayah Ranger District
90 Sloan Road
Franklin, North Carolina 28734
(828) 524-6441

Nantahala National Forest
Cheoah Ranger District
1133 Massey Branch Road
Robbinsville, North Carolina 28771
(828) 479-6487

# BENTON MACKAYE TRAIL

The Benton MacKaye Trail is what I imagine the Appalachian Trail was like many decades ago—a lesser-tamed path, steep in places, rough in spots, and still evolving. It is mostly well marked, less so in some locales—a mixture of occasional road walks and single-track footpaths treading along ridgelines and streams. Many sections of the Benton MacKaye Trail (BMT) have permanently fixed routes, while other sections are still being rerouted. The Benton MacKaye Trail shares other parallels with the Appalachian Trail. For starters, the trail's namesake, Benton MacKaye, was the man who actually conceived the idea of an "Appalachian Trail." The Benton MacKaye Trail starts at the same place as the AT, Springer Mountain in Georgia. It heads north through the Chattahoochee National Forest, like the AT, and crosses its more famous cousin a few times early during the 93-mile journey to its current terminus at the Ocoee River in Tennessee's Cherokee National Forest. Plans call for the BMT's extension north through the Cherokee to reach the Smoky Mountains National Park at Fontana Dam. It will then course through the Smokies to terminate at Davenport Gap, on the Smokies east end, covering a whopping 275 miles. I have no doubt this goal will be reached, as the Benton MacKaye Trail Association is doing a great job developing and maintaining this path.

Originally conceived in 1979, the Benton MacKaye (pronounced MAK-eye) Trail generally follows the western ridge of the Blue Ridge Mountains, which was the route for the Appalachian Trail as proposed by MacKaye. The BMT is a much-needed alternative to the overused Appalachian Trail for traversing North Georgia to the Smoky Mountains. The BMT has a much more remote sense to it than the AT. It is certainly less traveled. This is very evident where the AT and BMT intersect. The BMT is a narrow footpath, whereas the AT looks like a beaten down human highway in comparison.

The BMT isn't as easy to "use" as the AT. Often, the trail goes straight up and down the ridgeline, rather than gently switchbacking its way while changing elevations, which range from 1,500 feet to over

4,200 feet. There aren't conveniently located shelters; there aren't many marked side trails to water, supply points, or hostels. Campsites are much less frequent and not always obvious. The route can be overgrown. The diamond-shaped white blazes can be faint. However, on the plus side, these may be the very qualities you are looking for: a challenging route that takes effort to follow; a path where you must carry a lot of supplies, a trail with but one shelter and very few overcamped spots—in other words, a trail with solitude.

Currently, we have 90 excellent miles of hiking that make for a challenging weeklong-or-more journey or five ideal weekend backpacks. Starting at Springer Mountain, the trail swings along the escarpment of the Blue Ridge for a fine view, then descends into the Three Forks area in the Noontootla Creek Valley. It immediately works its way north into the John Dick Mountains before dropping to the Toccoa River. (The Toccoa River becomes the Ocoee River in Tennessee, the current terminus of the BMT, far from this crossing of the Toccoa.) Span the Toccoa on an elaborate suspension footbridge to walk up and over Toonowee Mountain before reaching Georgia Highway 60. Toonowee Mountain is your training ground—beyond GA 60 are two tough climbs up Wallalah Mountain and Licklog Mountain. Grab a view from Rhodes Mountain before descending to Skeenah Gap.

The trail treads over low, unsung mountains that show signs of a timbering past and little current visitation before dipping into Wilscot Gap. Here, the BMT makes a challenging pull up Tipton Mountain, then over Brawley Mountain before dropping to Garland Gap, a classic high-country saddle. From here, the BMT skirts around Garland Mountain and descends again to the Toccoa River, crossing this time on a road bridge. This bridge crossing precedes a road walk along Stanley Creek before the trail re-enters national-forest land with a bang, passing Fall Branch Falls and working its way up Rocky Mountain. Descend from this secluded mountaintop to Weaver Creek Road and head west, crossing US 76 to enter the Sisson Easement. The trail makes some unusual twists and turns here, as it wends its way northwest through a private mountain home development.

Beyond the Sisson Easement, the trail makes a bit of a road walk before re-entering national-forest land at Bushy Head Gap. From here to

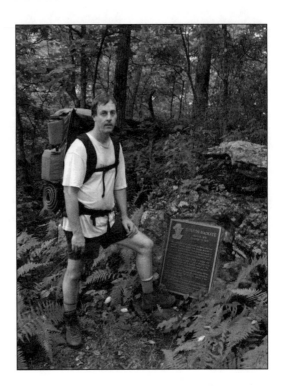

Benton MacKaye plaque
near Springer Mountain

its end at the Ocoee River, the Benton MacKaye Trail is at its best. Take
a rough and rugged ridge-running path that works up Bear Den Mountain and onward, finally descending to Hatley Gap, a good camping
spot. Just beyond the gap, the trail turns north and continues tracing
some of the most remote lands in Georgia, topping out on cool Flat Top
Mountain. From here, drop into the Jacks River watershed, where a dark
forest of hemlock and rhododendron awaits. Ahead lies the famed
Cohutta Wilderness. The trail reaches Hemp Top in the Cohutta, while
beelining north along the Blue Ridge to enter Tennessee's Cherokee
National Forest at Double Springs Gap.

Just across the state line lies another wilderness, Big Frog. Here, the
BMT reaches its high point, 4,224 feet, atop Big Frog Mountain. As it
keeps north, the trail cruises a ridgeline that avails numerous far-
reaching views before descending to West Prong Rough Creek. Finally,
the Benton MacKaye Trail leaves Big Frog Wilderness and works its way

north, dropping steeply into the Ocoee River gorge to end at Thunder Rock Campground.

Overnight camping opportunities on the BMT are limited. You must plan ahead for places to overnight on the dry ridges that can be short on flat ground and water. When seeking camp, water may be near, but no flat ground. Or a nice flat spot will be far from water. Backpackers usually camp at gaps on ridges or near the occasional stream. One trail shelter has been built on the Sisson Easement.

Hiking the Benton MacKaye Trail is a year-round proposition. Be apprised that winter extends much later in the North Georgia Mountains than many unfamiliar with the Southern Appalachians assume. Late spring and early summer are ideal times to hike. The BMT can be overgrown, warm, and relatively buggy in late summer. Conditions improve in fall, though this is generally when mountain springs are at their lowest flow. Regardless of the time of year, the BMT is nearly deserted during the week. Weekends see more hikers, especially around Springer Mountain and the Cohutta Wilderness.

There are a few resupply points along the Benton MacKaye Trail, though only one, a restaurant, is very convenient. Thunder Rock Campground, at the trail's northern terminus, makes for a safe end point with good parking. Even without supply runs, backpackers can carry enough food and gear for the entire outing from Springer Mountain to the Ocoee River. After hiking the Benton MacKaye Trail from end-to-end, I recommend the BMT experience over the Appalachian Trail experience in Georgia's Chattahoochee National Forest.

# Benton MacKaye Trail, Springer Mountain to Little Skeenah Creek

| | |
|---|---|
| **Length:** | 17.4 miles |
| **Trail Condition:** | Good |
| **Highs:** | Springer Mountain, views, Long Creek Falls, Toccoa River suspension bridge |
| **Lows:** | Potential crowds near Springer |
| **Season:** | Year-round; best during late spring, early summer, and fall |
| **Difficulty:** | Moderate to difficult |
| **Use:** | Heavy near Springer Mountain and Toccoa River, moderate elsewhere |
| **Tips:** | Leave Springer Mountain during the week if possible; if camping near Toccoa River, do so during the week |
| **Campsites:** | 2.2, 6.2, 8.6, 10.1, and 14.3 miles |

**SPRINGER MOUNTAIN TRAILHEAD:** From the point where US 76 and GA 52 cross near East Ellijay (76 overcomes 52 on an overpass), take GA 52 east for 4.8 miles to Big Creek Road. Turn left on Big Creek Road, and follow it for 12.5 miles to FR 42. Mount Pleasant Baptist Church is at the junction of FR 42 and Big Creek Road. Turn right on gravel FR 42 and follow it 6.8 miles to the Springer Mountain parking area on the left. From here, take the AT south, back across FR 42 for 0.7 miles to the signed left turn marking the beginning of the Benton MacKaye Trail.

**LITTLE SKEENAH CREEK TRAILHEAD:** From the junction of US 76 and GA 60 just east of Blue Ridge and northwest of Morgantown, head south on GA 60 for 13.7 miles and look for the brown hiker sign. If you pass Toccoa Bend Country Store on your right, you have gone 0.3 miles too far.

This trail segment marks the southern terminus of the Benton MacKaye Trail. Here, the BMT begins atop Springer Mountain, also the start of the Appalachian Trail. It immediately diverges from the AT, only to join the AT for two short sections en route to Three Forks, a pretty mountain valley. Here, the BMT turns northwest, running in conjunction with the Duncan Ridge Trail as it travels the ridgeline of the John Dick Mountains and descends to the Toccoa River. An attractive but potentially crowded campsite lies alongside this large mountain stream with angling opportunities. From here, the trail ascends Toonowee Mountain, then drops down to GA 60 near Little Skeenah Creek. Numerous camping opportunities are possible atop Springer Mountain: along a feeder stream of Chester Creek past Big Stamp Gap, down on Long Creek near Three Forks, at a gap above Mill Creek, at Bryson Gap, and along the Toccoa River.

❀    ❀    ❀

Since the beginning of the Benton MacKaye Trail is not directly accessible via the road, you must first hike a 0.7-miles section of the Appalachian Trail up Springer Mountain, starting at the FR 42 parking lot. Once you reach the intersection with the BMT, you can walk an additional 0.2 miles along the AT to reach the top of Springer Mountain. On the way to the top of Springer, pass the side trail to the Springer Mountain shelter and water source. This shelter has a loft, picnic table, and fire grate. A spring flows nearby. A plaque marking the trail and a view await at the top of the 3,782-foot mountain. Keep in mind that the 17.4-mile length of this section does not include the approach hike or the hike up to Springer, which together add an extra 1.1 miles to the hike.

Return to the intersection of the AT and the BMT to begin the Benton MacKaye Trail. The BMT is marked with diamond-shaped white blazes as it courses among young oaks growing over rock outcrops and ferns. At 0.1 miles, on the right, a plaque commemorates Benton MacKaye. Descend away from Springer Mountain as the bulk of the mountainside drops sharply to your right. At mile 1.4, a sign marks a side trail leading right, to a view. Here, on the edge of a steep rockface, look east toward Little Sal Mountain. The BMT continues its descent to reach FR 42 and Big Stamp Gap at mile 1.8. Cross the forest road, descend to and through the gap, entering a forest heavy with white pines. The trail curves back westward to cross a high-country stream cloaked in rhododendron at mile

2.2. Just past the crossing, on the right, is a small campsite. The fist-sized aromatic green plant lining the trail is galax. It was once heavily harvested for flower arrangements.

Ascend away from the stream over a small gap, then drop down to step over a couple of small streams and meet the Appalachian Trail at mile 3.1. Notice the difference in the treadways—the AT is much more heavily used. Continue forward as the two trails share the same path, making a pleasant forest cruise. At mile 3.3, the trail abruptly turns right. Dead ahead is FR 42. You have nearly circled back to your original parking area. Pass a flat where the Cross Trails shelter once stood. This area is too close to the forest road for good camping. Climb away from the shelter site to where the AT turns left at mile 3.9. Follow the BMT right and work your way down toward Three Forks on a mix of old roads and trails. The streams below become audible as the path passes under rhododendron tunnels before joining the AT a second time at mile 5.9. Here, the BMT turns right and runs in conjunction with the AT over Chester Creek (no camping allowed) on a footbridge and out to FR 58. Keep forward, crossing FR 58, and soon reach Long Creek. The twin trails ascend beneath tall white pines along Long Creek, where there are campsites.

Reach a three-way trail junction at mile 6.8. The AT continues forward while the Benton MacKaye Trail leaves left, now sharing the treadway with the Duncan Ridge Trail. (A separate side path leads sharp left a short piece to Long Creek Falls, which is worth the stop. The BMT/ Duncan Ridge Trail passes atop the falls before crossing Long Creek on a footbridge among towering hemlocks. Enter the intimate, attractive valley of a Long Creek feeder stream to ultimately climb away from the water and reach a wildlife clearing at mile 8.0. In summer tall grasses fill this clearing. Descend away from the clearing to reach a gap and a very small campsite at mile 8.6. Water can be found by heading northeast down the gap to the headwaters of Mill Creek.

The BMT continues north, heading toward the John Dick Mountains over a series of knobs in hickory-oak-maple woods with an understory of sassafras and wild azalea. After a long downhill switchback, reach Bryson Gap and a campground at mile 10.1. Several old roads cross this large campsite. Head right, east, down a side path to reach water. The BMT ascends away from the gap, skirting the west slope of the Little John Dick

Mountain while paralleling the Blue Ridge Wildlife Management Area boundary and offering some westward views along a bluffline. Reach Sapling Gap at mile 12.5, where you should notice several old roads. The main path is evident as it unevenly descends toward the Toccoa River, which is audible as the path crosses FR 333. Keep heading down among hemlock trees then veer left near the water. Dead ahead, at mile 14.3, is the surprisingly large and elaborate Toccoa River suspension footbridge. A spring and overused campsite lie on this side of the river and more campsites lie across the 265-foot span along the river.

The single-track BMT continues forward, crossing a closed forest road, and winds up the spine of Toonowee Mountain, cresting out at mile 15.0. Continue along the narrow ridgeline beneath oaks as it undulates for another 1.5 miles. Descend off the ridge to cross and parallel an intermittent streambed, then reach GA 60 and Little Skeenah Creek at mile 17.4. About 0.3 miles to your right (east) is a small grocery store with food and limited camping supplies.

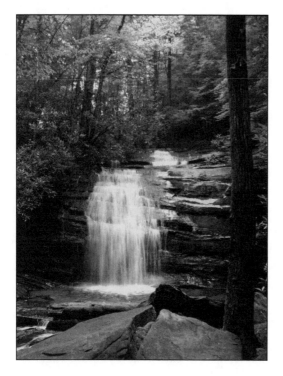

Long Creek Falls

# Benton MacKaye Trail, Little Skeenah Creek to Shallowford Bridge

| | |
|---|---|
| **Length:** | 18.8 miles |
| **Trail Condition:** | Good |
| **Highs:** | Some views, solitude |
| **Lows:** | Steep climbs straight up ridgelines |
| **Season:** | Year-round; best during late spring, early summer, and fall |
| **Difficulty:** | Difficult |
| **Use:** | Moderate to low |
| **Tips:** | Keep apprised of water supplies and water locations on trail |
| **Campsites :** | 3.8, 8.1, and 15.4 miles |

**LITTLE SKEENAH CREEK TRAILHEAD:** From the junction of US 76 and GA 60 just east of the town of Blue Ridge and northwest of Morgantown, head south on GA 60 for 13.7 miles and look for the brown hiker sign. If you pass Toccoa Bend Country Store on your right, you have gone 0.3 miles too far. There is limited parking along GA 60.

**SHALLOWFORD BRIDGE TRAILHEAD:** From Blue Ridge at the junction of US 76 and GA 5, head east on 76 for 0.8 miles and turn right on Windy Ridge Road. Follow Windy Ridge Road 0.1 miles to First Street at a T intersection. Turn left on First Street (toward Lake Blue Ridge) and follow it 0.1 miles to Aska Road. Turn right on Aska Road and follow it 8.4 miles to Shallowford Bridge, which will be on your left. Park in the gravel lot beside the Toccoa River.

This portion of the BMT has a challenging beginning, as it steeply climbs Wallalah Mountain, then descends, only to make another tough pull up Licklog Mountain. You'll stop short of the Rhodes Mountain summit where the Benton MacKaye and Duncan Ridge trails diverge. The Duncan Ridge Trail continues up, while the BMT drops northwest toward Skeenah Gap. The ascents become shorter as the path rolls over low, timbered ridgelines between Skeenah Gap and Wilscot Gap. Cross GA 60, then climb switchbacks up to Tipton Mountain. Drop to Ledford Gap only to climb Brawley Mountain, which has a fire tower that is closed to the public. The trail mostly descends from Brawley down to the Toccoa River and Shallowford Bridge, which is your route across the river.

Camping spots with water are located at a gap between Licklog and Rhodes Mountains at mile 3.8, at Payne Gap at mile 8.1, and at Garland Gap near Brawley Mountain at mile 15.4. Otherwise, water sources are infrequent and troublesome to reach; water from Little Skeenah Creek is not recommended for consumption.

❀    ❀    ❀

Leave GA 60 and immediately cross Little Skeenah Creek on a footbridge. Bisect a couple of old roads, then follow the undulating trail among tall white pines. Just when you begin to wonder about this supposed big climb, it begins, at mile 1.0, as the trail picks up a woods road heading straight up the ridgeline. Leave the roadbed and switchback uphill among boulders, where you can look south. Keep climbing to reach the top of Wallalah Mountain at mile 1.9. Immediately descend off the knob on a skinny ridgeline to make the gap between Wallalah and Licklog mountains. Ascend in fits and starts before nosing up the ridge to make a lungbuster of a climb and reach a small grassy clearing and the top of Licklog Mountain at mile 3.5. The BMT veers left, turning generally north, and drops off the east side of Licklog to reach a gap at mile 3.8. You'll find a campsite here as well as a water access path leading very steeply east off the ridgeline. The BMT descends a bit more before making the south flank of Rhodes Mountain. Just as the climb is getting rough, reach a trail junction at mile 4.4. Here, the Benton MacKaye mercifully drops off the west side of the ridge and the Duncan Ridge Trail keeps climbing Rhodes Mountain. (For a view, detour up the Duncan Ridge Trail another 0.1 miles, then look left, off the trail, for a rockface that looks out toward Wilscot Mountain.)

Descend the west slope of Rhodes Mountain and pick up an old roadbed in pine-oak woods. This roadbed has many earthen erosion barriers that give the mostly downhill path a roller coaster effect. At mile 5.7, come under a power line and veer left, paralleling the power line a short distance before turning right and taking a few steps up to reach Skeenah Gap. The BMT crosses Skeenah Gap Road and immediately passes through a series of white pine groves broken occasionally by young spindly woods, evidence of fairly recent logging. Wind mostly northward through low-slung hills. Work around an unnamed knob, making an abrupt right turn onto a woods road at mile 7.3. Keep north just a bit more before descending westward via a couple of switchbacks to reach Payne Gap at mile 8.1. Logging roads spur off in all directions at this camping flat. To reach water, head north out of Payne Gap and descend a draw to reach a seep. If you can't get water from the seep, keep tracing it downhill to reach a more substantial stream about 15 minutes from the gap. If you go this way, notice the rock walls of an old homesite near the stream. You could camp down here rather than in the gap.

The BMT continues west out of Payne Gap through young woods of tulip trees, oak, and maple. The young forest allows southward views of Licklog Mountain. Blackened bases of trees here are evidence of an old forest fire. Bisect FR 640-A at mile 9.0. Work your way up Deadennen Mountain, then switchback off the mountain to regain the ridgeline. Swing around the south side of Wilscot Mountain before passing wooden vehicle barriers at Wilscot Gap and GA 60 at mile 11.0. Across the road, to your left, is gated FR 45. Do not take this road. Instead, look right for a more overgrown gated road. Just near the overgrown gated road is the continuation of the BMT, now a single-track path. The trail wastes no time ascending Tipton Mountain. The BMT picks up a roadbed that winds among the arrow-straight gray trunks of tulip trees, which enjoy the moist northeast-facing slopes. On the right at mile 12.0, a spring drips water over a wide rockface. Keep switchbacking up the mountain, only to top out, passing a metal survey marker and curve around the steep north side of Tipton Mountain. As the path makes its way to the west side of the mountain, the trail becomes much rockier, offering views of Brawley Mountain and its signature fire tower. At mile 13.1, pass a side trail leading left to a wildlife clearing. Descend a few steps to reach another side trail leading right to a spring. Camping is not encouraged or recommended in the preceding wildlife clearing.

The BMT keeps forward to swing around Bald Top, which is recovering from logging, and reach FR 45 at ugly Ledford Gap, which is surrounded by ragged trees forming a low, thorny jungle. Turn right and walk FR 45 a few feet before re-entering the woods to begin the climb up

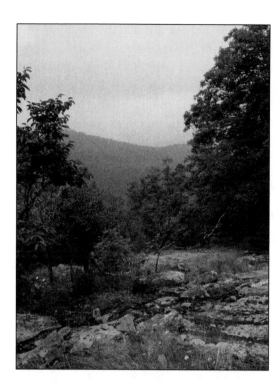

View from rock outcrop near
Rhodes Mountain

Brawley Mountain's northern slope. Pass by brushy young woods mixed
with some older oak trees on your way to the top of Brawley at mile
14.3, where you'll find a fire tower, a few outbuildings, and the end of
FR 45 on this 3,200-foot peak. While you might be tempted to climb the
fire tower, the absent bottom two rungs of the ladder prevent its use by
passersby. Turn right, away from the tower, and walk down FR 45 about
40 yards before turning right into the forest. Curve around Brawley on a
dug footbed, passing a level shelf with campsites but no water. Keep
switchbacking down to make Garland Gap at mile 15.4. This gap has a
flat spot for a camping and water access. Head right (north), down the
gap, to reach a spring.

Leave Garland Gap to follow the north slope of Garland Mountain
and pick up the ridgeline, stairstepping down. While descending this precipitous slope, you should hear the Toccoa River before the BMT reaches
Dial Road and a four-way gravel intersection at mile 17.0. Pick up the

trail on the other side of the intersection, and ascend westerly through pine woods toward Free Knob, before turning south to reach Shallowford Bridge Road and the Toccoa River at mile 18.3. Turn right on the road, passing numerous riverside houses to cross Shallowford Bridge at mile 18.8, reaching Aska Road and the end of this segment of the BMT. To the right, just down Aska Road, is a restaurant.

## Benton MacKaye Trail, Shallowford Bridge to Bushy Head Gap

| | |
|---|---|
| **Length:** | 19.4 miles |
| **Trail Condition:** | Good to fair |
| **Highs:** | Fall Branch Falls, Rocky Mountain, trail shelter |
| **Lows:** | Two long road walks |
| **Season:** | Year-round; best during late spring, early summer, and fall |
| **Difficulty:** | Moderate, except for climb of Rocky Mountain from Stanley Creek Road |
| **Use:** | Moderate |
| **Tips:** | Limited camping here; plan ahead. |
| **Campsites:** | 8.0, 9.6, and 14.6 miles |

**SHALLOWFORD BRIDGE TRAILHEAD:** From the town of Blue Ridge, where US 76 and GA 5 diverge, head east on US 76 for 0.8 miles and turn right on Windy Ridge Road. Follow Windy Ridge Road 0.1 miles to First Street at a T intersection. Turn left on First Street (toward Lake Blue Ridge) and follow it 0.1 miles to Aska Road. Turn right on Aska Road and follow it 8.4 miles to Shallowford Bridge, which will be on your left. Park in the gravel lot beside the Toccoa River.

**BUSHY HEAD GAP TRAILHEAD:** From the junction of US 76 and GA 5 in Ellijay, head north on US 76 for 10.6 miles to Gilmer CR 187. Turn left on CO 187 and follow it 2.7 miles to Boardtown Road. Veer right onto Boardtown Road and follow it 0.4 miles to Bushy Head Gap

Road. Turn left on Bushy Head Gap Road and follow it 1.8 miles to the top of the gap. Just past the gap, on the left, is a limited parking area at the beginning of FR 793.

Because of two long road walks, this part of the BMT will appeal mostly to end-to-end hikers. It really doesn't stand out on its own as a weekend hike, save for the portion over Rocky Mountain. Start on Aska Road at Shallowford Bridge, and walk to Stanley Creek Road. Trace Stanley Creek Road to enter National Forest land, making a splash of an entry at Fall Branch Falls. From the cascade, climb up Rocky Mountain in boulder-studded remote forestland, only to wind downhill, passing a small stream just before reaching Weaver Creek Road. Descend along Laurel Creek through a mountain home development to cross US 76 near Blue Ridge, Georgia, and enter another mountain home development, the Sisson property, where the trail takes roads and woods paths among the homes. A trail shelter is located on the Sisson property. Leave the Sisson development to reach Boardtown Road and make a last road walk to reach Bushy Head Gap and Chattahoochee National Forest.

Campsites with water are limited in this section; they are found at mile 8.0, the gap north of Rocky Mountain, mile 9.6, the creek just before Weaver Creek Road, and the trail shelter on the Sisson property at mile 14.6. Other than that, you will have to carry your water to a campsite of your choosing.

❋    ❋    ❋

Leave Shallowford Bridge and head southwest on Aska Road, following the Toccoa River downstream. Walk past a restaurant on your left, then pass a piped spring coming in from the hillside at 0.3 miles. Soon pass another restaurant on the right with very limited supplies, then turn left onto paved Stanley Creek Road at 0.4 miles. The occasional diamond trail markers are posted along the road. At mile 3.1, the pavement ends. Keep forward, spanning Fall Branch on a road bridge. Immediately turn right onto an old woods road and begin ascending steeply along the rhododendron-lined creek. You are now in the Chattahoochee National Forest. At mile 3.6, a side trail leads right to the three-tiered Fall Branch Falls, which can be viewed from a wooden platform. The BMT leaves the old woods road just a bit past the falls, turning left onto a foot trail. The trail swings around to a ridgeline and heads up Rocky Mountain into a section of woods once ravaged by fire. In points, the trail itself was used as a firebreak, resulting in woods of different ages on either side of the path.

At mile 4.6, the Stanley Gap Trail joins the BMT from the left. The two trails continue forward together as they switchback up and curve around Rocky Mountain. Tree types change from pine to birch as the path winds around the peak. Higher up the mountain are vast fern fields broken by boulder outcrops. At mile 6.3, regain the ridgecrest, having bypassed the mountain summit. Undulate along the ridgeline to reach a second junction at mile 6.7. Here, the Stanley Gap Trail heads right toward Deep Gap. The BMT keeps forward and soon drops down, passing a side trail marked by a pile of stones at mile 7.6. This side trail leads right, dropping steeply for about 100 yards to reach a spring. At mile 8.0, reach the gap between Rocky Mountain and Scroggin Knob. It is level enough for camping but is rarely used. Water can be had from the spring 0.4 mile back or by dropping right (north) from the trail to a spring-branch of Stillhouse Creek.

To continue, ascend away from the gap and soon top out on Scroggin Knob, where a dry, north-looking campsite lies. Drop off the ridge to take switchbacks down through dry pine wood coves, eventually reaching a feeder branch of Laurel Creek at mile 9.6. Just over a small hill lies a second branch. This area, although near Weaver Creek Road, does have flat areas for camping and is on National Forest land. The BMT turns away from the feeder branch, meanders through young pine woods, and emerges onto gravel Weaver Creek Road at mile 9.7.

The BMT follows the gravel road left, passing though fields and woods to cross Laurel Creek. The trail then runs downhill, mostly through a mountain housing development. Follow the blazes carefully to reach US 76 at mile 12.8. Cross the divided highway and walk left along the road for 150 yards to re-enter the woods beside a fence line. Do not cross the metal fence, but rather run along it a bit until you can climb into the Sisson Easement. Circle around a small knob to reach Cherry Log Creek. Walk beneath the covered road bridge and keep forward to reach railroad tracks at mile 13.2. Do not cross the tracks; instead, turn left and parallel the tracks a short distance, then cross the tracks and enter a small streamshed, Sisson Creek.

After passing a waterfall, you'll come to a development road. From here to the end of the section, the trail alternately follows roads flanked with modern log cabins and wooded strips between cabins. As the development continues, the exact path of the BMT will change, but for now, it overlooks Cherry Lake from a platform near the lake dam. Keep a close eye on the white diamond blazes as the trail comes alongside a feeder branch of Sisson Creek to reach a trail shelter at mile 14.6. The shelter is walled on three sides and has wooden bunks and a fire grate. The feeder branch is the water source.

Beyond the shelter, the BMT passes Indian Rock Lake beneath another covered bridge, then soon leaves left on an old road. Climb the roadbed, passing a blue-blazed trail at mile 15.0 (the former path of the BMT before it was relocated), which heads left toward Lucius Road. The current BMT climbs toward Patterson Mountain and keeps northwest in woods to descend along a small stream, reaching Boardtown Road near the Fannin-Gilmer county line at mile 16.6. Turn left on Boardtown Road and follow it southwest for one mile to Bushy Head Road. Turn right on Bushy Head Road, immediately spanning Boardtown Creek on the paved road bridge. Bushy Head Mountain is visible ahead and to the right. Keep rising to meet Bushy Head Gap, just past Cub Trail Road, at mile 19.4, to end this portion of the Benton MacKaye Trail.

# Benton MacKaye Trail, Bushy Head Gap to Watson Gap

| | |
|---|---|
| **Length:** | 17.4 miles |
| **Trail Condition:** | Good to fair |
| **Highs:** | Solitude, Flat Top Mountain area and South Fork Jacks River |
| **Lows:** | Poorly marked overgrown trail in places |
| **Season:** | Year-round; best during late spring, early summer, and fall |
| **Difficulty:** | Moderate to strenuous |
| **Use:** | Low |
| **Tips:** | Many old logging roads, stay with white diamond blazes and backtrack if you lose blazes |
| **Campsites:** | 5.0, 3.0, 9.9, and 15.0 miles |

**BUSHY HEAD GAP TRAILHEAD:** From the junction of US 76 and GA 5 in Ellijay, head north on US 76 for 10.6 miles to Gilmer CR 187. Turn left on CR 187 and follow it 2.7 miles to Boardtown Road. Veer right onto Boardtown Road and follow it 0.4 miles to Bushy Head Gap Road. Turn left on Bushy Head Gap Road and follow it 1.8 miles to the top of the gap. Just past the gap, on the left is a limited parking area at the beginning of FR 793. The Benton MacKaye Trail starts just beyond the top of the gap.

**WATSON GAP TRAILHEAD:** From Blue Ridge, where US 76 and GA 5 diverge, head north on US 76 for 3.7 miles to Old SR 2. A sign will say "Old S. R. 2." Turn left here and follow Old SR 2 for 10.6 miles to Watson Gap, located at the intersection with FR 64 and FR 22. The Benton MacKaye Trail heads up FR 22 from the gap.

This portion of the Benton MacKaye Trail traverses some of the wildest land in the state of Georgia. You'll leave Bushy Head Gap and travel southwest along a rugged ridgeline to Hatley Gap. Keep southwest a bit more while ascending Fowler Mountain. From here, the trail turns north and begins heading to the high country of Flat Top Mountain. The BMT then descends to Dyer Gap and an old mountain cemetery. The path keeps dropping to meet South Fork Jacks River amid a forest of hemlock and rhododendron. It traces South Fork Jacks River, a quality trout stream, then takes old forest roads to reach to Watson Gap.

This forgotten section of the Chattahoochee National Forest oozes solitude. The few camping spots with water are good ones, located at Hatley Gap at mile 5.3 near Fowler Mountain, near a wildlife clearing on Flat Top Mountain at mile 9.9, and down along South Fork Jacks River at mile 15.0.

❀　　❀　　❀

Start this portion of the Benton MacKaye Trail by heading west from Bushy Head Gap on a dug foot trail that cuts into the woods. Follow around the northeast side of Bear Den Mountain in a laurel thicket to pick up an old woods road at 0.6 miles. Switchback up Bear Den Mountain with obscured views to the north. At mile 1.8, an unmaintained trail leaves right. Descend to reach Hudson Gap and FR 793 at mile 2.7. The BMT follows the forest road just a few feet, then re-enters the woods. Tack south-to-southeast while climbing the ridgeline with hemlocks growing about. The walking is mostly easy as it works around ridges into gaps and back around ridges, on and off old logging grades. The BMT drifts into McKenny Gap at mile 4.1. This small gap is grassy and has several old roads spurring off it.

From the gap, the BMT stays on the steep south side of a high knob. The trail regains the ridgecrest before passing a spring branch on trail-right at mile 5.2. This is a good water source for camping at Hatley Gap, located at mile 5.3. Wide Hatley Gap is grown up with blackberries, locust, and tulip trees, but still offers grassy and wooded locales for overnighting. Campers can also keep forward 0.1 miles beyond the gap to obtain water at a spring flowing off Fowler Mountain.

Beyond Hatley Gap, the trail descends a bit more before switchbacking up Fowler Mountain on a footpath. Soon, pass a spring branch, then rise among attractive coves before regaining the ridgeline at mile 6.1. Top out on Fowler Mountain at mile 6.9 and turn north to follow the western edge of the Cohutta Wildlife Management Area.

The section between Fowler Mountain and Dyer Gap is the least trammeled slice of the BMT, remaining above 3,000 feet until Dyer Gap. The presence of trailside cherry trees is indicative of the higher elevation. The path, a single-track trail often overlain on old logging grades, very well may be overgrown in late summer. Leaving Fowler Mountain, the trail passes over numerous low knobs, making a pleasant forest cruise, before dropping down via switchbacks to Halloway Gap at mile 8.8. Climb out of the gap, heading for Flat Top Mountain. Dip down and come near a stream on trail-left, just before reaching a wildlife clearing at mile 9.9. There are campsites in the woods bordering the clearing. Make an abrupt right turn at clearing, picking up an old road and resuming the climb.

The BMT soon leaves left away from the road and continues as a single-track path to drop down to several small rhododendron-cloaked streamlets feeding South Fork Jacks River. The heavy growth and sloped land are not favorable for camping. Rise away from the watershed, making for the top of Flat Top Mountain, passing near another wildlife clearing on trail-right. Level out and hike by a huge oak in a clearing. Just beyond here, at mile 11.6, is the site of the old Flat Top fire tower, which once stood on this 3,732-foot peak. The concrete pillars are all that remain of the tower.

The BMT continues north, descending off the knob in switchbacks on the rocky northwest side of the knob. There are occasional views to the west of rampart-like Cohutta Mountain. At mile 12.8, emerge onto FR 64-A. Turn left onto the gated dirt road and descend to reach FR 64 and Dyer Gap at mile 13.0. To your right is the Dyer Cemetery. Take time to visit this historic place of rest. It has old graves as well as new graves.

From the gap, the BMT turns left on FR 64, moving away from the cemetery, and heads west for a bit. Turn right, leaving the road behind, to drop into the South Fork Jacks River watershed and a dark forest of hemlock and rhododendron. Soon the waters gather in the hollow forming the river. The BMT meets the South Fork Jacks River Trail at mile 13.6 and turns right, working through woods on the edge of a large, open, beaver-created wetland on trail-left. The South Fork reappears below the wetland and soon becomes pinched in. Look left into the woodland for occasional, though not plentiful, riverside campsites as the trail winds in and out of small coves that feed more water in the river. The main river is good trout habitat. Reach a trail junction in Rich Cove at mile 15.2. The South Fork Jacks River Trail keeps forward while the BMT turns right, away from the river and up a hollow on an old forest road that is in the process of becoming forested itself. The canopy is often open overhead and ragged trees such as sumac are invading the area. The path eventually leaves the road and traces a pine-oak ridgeline. It works down to reach Watson Gap, Old SR 2, and the end of this segment of the Benton MacKaye Trail at mile 17.4.

## Benton MacKaye Trail, Watson Gap to Ocoee River

| | |
|---|---|
| **Length:** | 20.0 miles |
| **Trail Condition:** | Good |
| **Highs:** | Cohutta Wilderness, Big Frog Wilderness, highest point on BMT |
| **Lows:** | Potentially overgrown trail between FR 45 and Thunder Rock Campground |
| **Season:** | Year-round; best during late spring, early summer, and fall |
| **Difficulty:** | Moderate south-to-north |
| **Use:** | Moderate except in Cohutta Wilderness |
| **Tips:** | Trail not blazed in wilderness areas |
| **Campsites:** | 0.8, 2.1, 8.7, 9.6, 9.9, 15.4, and 20 miles |

**WATSON GAP TRAILHEAD:** From Blue Ridge, Georgia, where US 76 and GA 5 diverge, head north on US 76 for 3.7 miles to Old SR 2. A sign will say "Old SR 2." Turn left here and follow Old SR 2 for 10.6 miles to Watson Gap, located at the intersection with FR 64 and FR 22. The Benton MacKaye Trail heads up FR 22 from the gap.

**OCOEE RIVER TRAILHEAD:** From the junction of US 64 and US 64 Bypass, just east of Cleveland, Tennessee, take US 64 east for 26 miles to the right turn at Ocoee Dam #3 and Thunder Rock Campground. Turn right and cross the dam to turn right into Thunder Rock Campground. The Benton MacKaye trailhead is near campsite #T 24, toward the back of the campground. Trailhead parking is near the front of the campground across from the fee station.

The final portion of the BMT is it's finest. Leave Watson Gap and enter the Cohutta Wilderness. The path dips down to a couple of high elevation streams before regaining the Blue Ridge and heading north on a wide, old forest road, easily gaining elevation to peak out near Hemp Top, an old fire tower site. The trail drops down to enter Tennessee at Double Springs Gap, only to make a tough pull up Big Frog Mountain and into the Big Frog Wilderness. Reach the highest point of the BMT atop Big Frog, where yellow birch trees grow that favor the cool country farther north. The path then picks up a spindly ridgeline offering views both east and west among rock outcrops framed in grass and stunted trees. Keep working down to meet West Fork Rough Creek and travel along this small trout stream only to climb away and enter a network of multi-use trails emanating from the Ocoee River Whitewater Center. The well-blazed BMT remains easy to follow as it makes a final descent into the Ocoee River gorge and Thunder Rock Campground. Be apprised that the Benton MacKaye Trail is not blazed in either the Cohutta or Big Frog wildernesses, though it is signed at most trail junctions.

Campsites with water are ample and located along Mill Creek just north of Watson Gap at 0.8 miles; in Peter Cove just as the trail enters the Cohutta Wilderness at 2.1 miles; and at Double Springs Gap at the Tennessee-Georgia line at mile 8.7. In Tennessee, there are campsites at a gap just south of Big Frog Mountain at mile 9.6; on top of Big Frog Mountain at mile 9.9; along West Fork Rough Creek at mile 15.4; and at Thunder Rock Campground at trail's end, mile 20.0.

❀   ❀   ❀

Leave the parking area at Watson Gap and walk north on narrow FR 22 toward Dally Gap. Follow the road 0.3 miles and look for the BMT making an acute left turn off the forest road. The trail rises briefly then dips down to cross Mill Creek in a flat good for camping at 0.8 miles. Pick up an old rhododendron-shaded road, flanked by a rusty wire fence as it runs along Mill Branch. Step over a feeder branch of Mill Creek, then make an abrupt left, and ascend along the feeder branch.

The trail leaves the watershed to enter the Cohutta Wilderness along a low ridge at mile 1.5. Drop down in a hemlock forest to reach the stream of Peter Cove and a campsite at mile 2.1. Step over the stream and descend along the watercourse to meet Bear Branch at mile 2.4. Here, the path climbs away from the water to the intersection with the Jacks River Trail. The BMT runs in conjunction with the Jacks River Trail a short distance before heading left to climb a dry cove in a holly grove. The single-track trail winds mostly upward in pretty pine-oak woods to regain the Blue Ridge, then makes a short descent to meet the Hemp Top Trail in Spanish Oak Gap at mile 4.2. Turn left, as the Benton MacKaye Trail now runs in conjunction with the Hemp Top Trail, and continue north along the Blue Ridge, following the route of a closed forest road.

The wide roadbed makes for easy walking and before you know it, the BMT intersects the Penitentiary Gap Trail, at mile 5.6 near Rockwall Gap. Don't turn left, but continue north on the roadbed, passing rock cuts where the stone was blasted away to make the roadbed leading to Hemp Top. Grab occasional views of the Cohutta Wilderness to the west as the trail moderately ascends to meet the west side of 3,580-foot Hemp Top at mile 7.4. The trail leaves the recovering area and descends along a footpath to meet a much smaller woods road. The trail keeps north and pleasantly drifts down to Double Springs Gap and the Tennessee state line at mile 8.7. True to the gap's name, springs emanate from both the east and west side of the trail. There are two campsites located at this 3,200-foot gap: one just among the white pines and another in a small, sheltered flat to the east of the gap.

The BMT leaves the gap and passes a sign welcoming hikers into Tennessee's Cherokee National Forest. And what a welcome you receive—a terribly steep, 1,000-foot climb up Big Frog. Make the ascent to meet the Licklog Trail at mile 9.3. Veer left, as the BMT now runs in conjunction with the Licklog Trail. The climb moderates and passes a gap with camping. A spring is located down the draw to the north.

Ascend away from the gap to pass a deep, rocked-in spring on trail-left that can go dry in fall. Shortly after the spring, reach the top of Big Frog (4,224 feet) at mile 9.9. A trail junction and small, grassy clearing with a campsite are also here. Notice the surrounding yellow birch trees with their horizontal, peeling bark; the lands below them are too warm or dry to sustain them.

Straight ahead, the Wolf Ridge Trail begins, and soon leads to a small outcrop with a view. The BMT, however, veers right, now running in conjunction with the Big Frog Trail down Fork Ridge. This is a moderate descent with occasional views of the Tennessee mountains as the ridgeline narrows. The path steepens at some switchbacks. At mile 11.3, the trail runs along a narrow rocky ridgecrest that avails great views of East Fork Rough Creek valley, Licklog Ridge, and the lowlands in the distance. Just past here, the BMT meets the obscure Barkleggin Trail, which comes in sharply from the left and is marked by a pile of rocks. The BMT continues forward and swings around the west side of Chimneytop, then straddles a spindly ridge with many views and rock outcrops.

At mile 12.0, the BMT meets the Fork Ridge Trail and the Big Frog Trail leaves to the left. The BMT follows the Fork Ridge Trail forward and down the ridgeline. The trail continues to descend, winding through two small dry coves with Fraser magnolias before dipping off the east side of the ridge in a gap. The footbed is narrow here. The BMT regains the crest of Fork Ridge just before meeting the Rough Creek Trail in a T intersection at mile 13.8. The BMT leaves left, now running in conjunction with the Rough Creek Trail. Descend into moist forest to reach West Fork Rough Creek at mile 14.4. The clear mountain stream can be crossed without getting wet during times of normal flow. Climb away from the stream and pick up a forest road that was closed when Big Frog Wilderness was created in 1984. An old culvert and broken road bridge remain to the left.

At a rock cairn, The BMT turns right (north), leaving the Rough Creek Trail to continue westward. The BMT keeps forward on the old road and heads downstream along West Fork Rough Creek, now running in conjunction with the West Fork Rough Creek Trail. Cross the stream twice more, where the remains of old culverts still lie about the crossings. Beyond the last crossing, look for a couple of flats suitable for camping. Toward the end of the walk, the trail doubles as the wilderness boundary, with the Big Frog Wilderness on trail-right and undesignated forestland on trail-left. Leave the roadbed at a second rock cairn at mile 15.6. Here, the BMT, once again blazed, climbs along a small branch to pick up a seeded-over roadbed and reach FR 221 at mile 16.6.

Look across the gravel road, left, for a gated forest road descending away from FR 221. This is old FR 45. Pass around the metal gate and drop into the Little Gassaway Creek watershed with fairly large tulip trees. At mile 17.1, reach a three-way intersection. Here, the BMT Trail leaves left on a single-track path that follows the closed forest road. Work down to Little Gassaway Creek, spanning it on a footbridge. Turn uphill at a feeder branch on a broken-canopied trail, and circumvent an earthen vehicle barrier just before reaching current FR 45 on a curve at mile 18.4. Cross the forest road and keep forward, passing a sign indicating Thunder Rock Campground ahead. The BMT now runs in conjunction with the Thunder Rock Trail. The footbed narrows as it stays above FR 45 and passes a few gaps as it heads north. The Ocoee River becomes audible, then the BMT makes several switchbacks to enter the gorge of the Ocoee River. Reach the Ocoee River at mile 19.8, cross a wooden bridge near the river and keep upstream to enter Thunder Rock Campground and the current northern terminus of the BMT at mile 20.0.

## Benton MacKaye Trail Log

### SPRINGER MOUNTAIN TO LITTLE SKEENAH CREEK

| | | |
|---|---|---|
| 0.0 | 93.0 | BMT leaves from AT 0.7 miles from FR 42 near top of Springer Mountain |
| 0.1 | 92.9 | Benton MacKaye memorial plaque |
| 1.4 | 91.6 | Spur trail leaves right to view |
| 1.8 | 91.2 | Pass through Big Stamp Gap, cross FR 42 |
| 2.2 | 90.8 | High country stream, small campsite |
| 3.1 | 89.9 | Intersect the AT and again in 0.6 miles |
| 5.9 | 87.1 | Converge with the AT to cross Chester Creek on a footbridge, cross FR 58 |
| 6.8 | 86.2 | Trail junction, Long Creek Falls spur trail, AT and BMT diverge, BMT runs in conjunction with Duncan Ridge Trail |
| 8.0 | 85.0 | Reach wildlife clearing after steep ascent |
| 8.6 | 84.4 | Very small campsite in gap near headwaters of Mill Creek |
| 10.1 | 82.9 | Bryson Gap, campsite, and water |
| 12.5 | 80.5 | Sapling Gap, descend toward Toccoa River |
| 14.3 | 78.7 | Span Toccoa River on elaborate suspension bridge, campsites nearby |

## Benton MacKaye Trail Log *(continued)*

| | | |
|---|---|---|
| **15.0** | **78.0** | Crest of Toonowee Mountain, undulate along ridgeline |
| **17.4** | **75.6** | Reach GA 60, cross Little Skeenah Creek Little Skeenah Creek to Shallowford Bridge |
| **18.4** | **74.6** | Trail begins steep ascent of Wallalah Mountain |
| **19.3** | **73.7** | Crest out on Wallalah Mountain, descend to gap, then ascend Licklog Mountain |
| **20.9** | **72.1** | Crest out on Licklog Mountain |
| **21.2** | **71.8** | Reach gap with campsite and side trail to water, ascend toward Rhodes Mountain |
| **21.8** | **71.2** | BMT and Duncan Ridge trails diverge, BMT descends left toward Skeenah Gap |
| **23.1** | **69.9** | Come under power line then reach Skeenah Gap and cross paved Skeenah Gap Road, keep north in low-slung hills |
| **25.5** | **67.5** | Reach Payne Gap, with campsite and water |
| **26.4** | **66.6** | Cross FR 640-A, work up Deadennen Mountain |

### SHALLOWFORD BRIDGE TO BUSHY HEAD GAP

| | | |
|---|---|---|
| **28.4.** | **64.6** | Reach Wilscot Gap and GA 60. Cross GA 60 and ascend Tipton Mountain |
| **29.4** | **63.6** | Pass by spring on trail-right, keep ascending |
| **30.5** | **62.5** | Side trail leads left to wildlife clearing; spring just a bit down BMT on right. Work around Bald Top and descend to Ledford Gap. Ascend Brawley Mountain |
| **31.7** | **61.3** | Crest out on 3,200-foot Brawley Mountain and descend toward Garland Gap |
| **32.8** | **60.2** | Reach Garland Gap, with flat area for camping and spring to right of trail |
| **34.4** | **58.6** | Intersect Dial Road after stairstepping down from Garland Mountain |
| **35.7** | **57.3** | Reach Shallowford Bridge Road along Toccoa River |
| **36.2** | **56.8** | Cross Shallowford Bridge on Toccoa River, turn right onto Aska Road |

### SHALLOWFORD BRIDGE TO BUSHY HEAD GAP

| | | |
|---|---|---|
| **36.5** | **56.5** | Pass piped spring along Aska Road |
| **36.6** | **56.4** | Turn left onto paved Stanley Gap Road |
| **39.3** | **53.7** | Leave road and turn right into national-forest land, ascending along Fall Branch |
| **39.5** | **53.5** | Side trail leads right to Fall Branch Falls, begin ascent of Rocky Mountain |
| **40.5** | **52.5** | Intersect Stanley Gap Trail, which runs in conjunction with BMT |

## Benton MacKaye Trail Log *(continued)*

| | | |
|---|---|---|
| **42.6** | **50.4** | Stanley Gap Trail leaves right for Deep Gap; BMT keeps forward and descends |
| **43.7** | **49.3** | Pile of stones marks side trail leading right to spring |
| **44.1** | **48.9** | Reach gap between Rocky Mountain and Scroggin Knob, potential camping |
| **45.7** | **47.3** | Reach feeder branches of Laurel Creek, potential camping |
| **45.8** | **47.2** | Intersect Weaver Creek Road, leave left down gravel road, soon crossing Laurel Creek and passing beside private mountain homes |
| **48.9** | **44.1** | Cross busy US 76, turn left, and walk along road, soon entering Sisson Easement |
| **49.3** | **43.7** | Span covered bridge over Cherry Log Creek, turn left before railroad tracks, and begin winding through mountain home development |
| **50.7** | **42.3** | Reach trail shelter beside small stream, emerge to cross second covered bridge |
| **51.1** | **41.9** | Trail junction, old BMT leaves left for Lucius Road, newer BMT continues in easement on woods and road toward Patterson Mountain |
| **52.7** | **40.3** | Intersect Boardtown Road near Fannin-Gilmer county line; turn left on Boardtown Road |
| **53.7** | **39.3** | Reach Bushy Head Gap Road, turn right and ascend toward Bushy Head Gap |
| **55.6** | **37.4** | BMT leaves road at gap just beyond Cub Trail Road, enters national-forest land and ascends Bear Den Mountain |

## BUSHY HEAD GAP TO WATSON GAP

| | | |
|---|---|---|
| **56.2** | **36.8** | Intersect woods road and keep climbing |
| **58.3** | **34.7** | Reach Hudson Gap and FR 793 |
| **59.7** | **33.3** | Reach McKenny Gap, work around left side of steep ridge |
| **60.8** | **32.2** | Pass spring in draw on trail-right |
| **60.9** | **32.1** | Reach Hatley Gap with good camping then ascend toward Fowler Mountain |
| **61.0** | **32.0** | Pass spring on Fowler Mountain |
| **62.5** | **30.5** | Top out on Fowler Mountain, trail turns north on dim track |
| **64.4** | **28.6** | Reach Halloway Gap after descending switchback |
| **65.5** | **27.5** | Pass stream near wildlife clearing, campsites near clearing |
| **67.2** | **25.8** | Top out on 3,732-foot Flat Top Mountain at old fire tower site, descend toward Dyer Gap |
| **68.4** | **24.6** | Emerge onto FR 64-A, turn left, and descend |
| **68.6** | **24.4** | Reach FR 64 at Dyer Gap. Dyer Cemetery to right, BMT turns left on FR 64, soon turns right into woods, and descends toward South Fork Jacks River |

## Benton MacKaye Trail Log *(continued)*

| | | |
|---|---|---|
| **69.2** | **23.8** | Intersect South Fork Jacks River Trail, keep right, campsites downstream along river |
| **70.8** | **22.2** | Leave South Fork Jacks River in Rich Cove and ascend on old forest roads toward Watson Gap |
| **73.0** | **20.0** | Reach Watson Gap, head north on FR 22 toward Dally Gap |

### WATSON GAP TO OCOEE RIVER

| | | |
|---|---|---|
| **73.3** | **19.7** | Turn acutely left away from FR 22 and descend toward Mill Creek |
| **73.8** | **19.2** | Reach Mill Creek, potential camping. Ascend toward Cohutta Wilderness |
| **74.5** | **18.5** | Enter Cohutta Wilderness, then descend to Peter Cove |
| **75.1** | **17.9** | Cross stream in Peter Cove, campsite |
| **75.4** | **17.6** | Step over Bear Branch in rhododendron thicket |
| **17.3** | | Intersect and turn right on Jacks River Trail, then soon turn left and ascend toward Blue Ridge |
| **77.5** | **15.5** | Meet Hemp Top Trail in Spanish Oak Gap, turn left and follow wide former forest road, now in conjunction with Hemp Top Trail |
| **78.9** | **14.1** | Intersect Penitentiary Branch Trail which leaves left; BMT keeps forward |
| **80.7** | **12.3** | Reach 3,580-foot Hemp Top; descend toward Double Springs Gap |
| **82.0** | **11.0** | Reach Double Springs Gap and Tennessee state line. Camping and water here. Enter Cherokee National Forest and Big Frog Wilderness, steep ascent |
| **82.6** | **10.4** | Intersect Licklog Trail, keep left |
| **83.2** | **9.8** | Reach top of 4,220-foot Big Frog Mountain after passing spring. Camping atop mountain, veer right in conjunction with Big Frog Trail |
| **84.6** | **8.4** | Rocky ridgecrest avails great views |
| **85.3** | **7.7** | Keep forward in conjunction with Fork Ridge Trail as Big Frog Trail leaves left |
| **86.9** | **6.1** | Reach T intersection, BMT turns left in conjunction with Rough Creek Trail |
| **87.5** | **5.5** | Step over West Fork Rough Creek and reach old forest road, turn right, now in conjunction with West Fork Trail, campsites down trail in flats along West Fork |
| **88.7** | **4.3** | Blazed BMT leaves left away from West Fork and ascends |
| **89.6** | **3.4** | Reach FR 221; descend along gated old FR 45 |
| **90.1** | **2.9** | Reach three-way trail intersection; keep left, cross Little Gassaway Creek |

## Benton MacKaye Trail Log *(continued)*

**91.4** **1.6** Reach FR 45, cross forest road and straddle ridge to reach Ocoee River gorge, descend into gorge via switchbacks

**92.8** **0.2** Come alongside Ocoee River, head upstream

**93.0** **0.0** Reach Thunder Rock Campground and current trail terminus

## Benton MacKaye Trail Information

Benton MacKaye Trail Association
P.O. Box 53271
Atlanta, Georgia 30355-1271
www.bmta.org

Chattahoochee National Forest
1755 Cleveland Highway
Gainesville, Georgia 30501
(770) 297-3000
www.fs.fed.us/conf/

Chattahoochee National Forest
Toccoa Ranger District
6050 Appalachian Highway
Blue Ridge, Georgia 30513
(706) 632-3031

Chattahoochee National Forest
Cohutta Ranger District
3941 Highway 76
Chatsworth, Georgia 30705
(706) 695-6736

Cherokee National Forest
P.O. Box 2010
Cleveland, Tennessee 37320
(423) 476-9700
www.southernregion.fs.fed.us/
    cherokee

Cherokee National Forest
Ocoee-Hiwassee Ranger District
Route 1, Box 348D
Benton, Tennessee 37307
(423) 338-5201

# BLACK CREEK TRAIL

The Black Creek Trail (BCT) is not only the apex of hiking in the Magnolia State, it is also one of the finest hiking trails in the Southeastern United States. This path makes a 41-mile trek through rich, diverse woodlands of the De Soto National Forest that veil the corridor of the Black Creek watershed. Black Creek itself is so eye appealing as to be a federally designated wild and scenic river, the only one in the state of Mississippi. It is along this creek that much of the trail travels, offering views of the tea-colored waters that contrast with burning white sandbars, banked against verdant green forests so thick as to seem impenetrable. But somehow, the Black Creek Trail works its way up the river valley, not only along the clear waterway, but also over innumerable side creeks, spanned by boardwalks and footbridges. There is still water back here, too, where cypress and gum trees emerge from the dark swamps, adding to the junglesque character of the Black Creek watershed. It's not all water and deep woods in the Gulf Coast Plain of Mississippi—there are also open pine forests that reach for the sky in the hill country that abuts the Black Creek floodplain. These forests offer a contrast to the rich woodlands along the creek.

The Black Creek Trail starts at Fairley Bridge Landing, on the lower end of Black Creek. The net elevation gain to the upper end is only 50 feet, but don't expect a flat road walk. Leaving the trailhead behind, the path immediately turns away from Black Creek and heads through lush woods and wetlands, spanning the first of over 80 boardwalks and footbridges. The trail then heads for the Red Hills. These surprisingly steep hills are cut by swift sand-bottomed streams. The trail climbs up and down these heavily vegetated rises where interesting species such as the big leaf magnolia, with tropical looking leaves in excess of 25 inches in length, thrive. Piney woods reign on the hilltops. Just as you begin to wonder what happened to Black Creek, the trail returns streamside, where sandbars are accessible for relaxing, or camping, or as a place to lay your pack while you dip in the refreshing waters.

The trail quickly returns to hill country before entering the Black Creek Wilderness, a special protected swath of the De Soto National Forest. Wander through oak woodlands before coming alongside Mill Creek, with its small waterfalls heading noisily for Black Creek. Thus begins the first lengthy stretch of wandering in the Black Creek floodplain. It continues, sometimes along the river, where the loud slap of a beavertail startles trail travelers who regularly span footbridges over streambeds, wet and dry, and sometimes up and down little valleys where deer furtively feed in morning and evening. Also down here are the swamps. These still places are broken only by birdsong, the croaking of frogs, the throng of insects in the night, and the occasional footfall of a hiker walking by. The trail then circles Beaverdam Creek, a small blackwater stream entering the wilderness from the west.

The path leaves the wilderness and works its way along the edge of Black Creek, where bottomland hardwood forests grow to the edge of the river, passing many accessible sandbars. It then heads to the margin of land where the floodplain meets the hills, winding north and west on a plethora of overgrown woods roads, before returning to a tortuously winding stretch of Black Creek. Here, the path seeks high ground among the dense concentration of wetlands, bottoms, and swamps in a thick forest that keeps midday dark. The blindingly bright white sandbars of the stream jump out at you after a stint in the dim forest.

Seemingly just for contrast, the trail makes another run for the hills before coming to the longest riverside stretch of them all. Here, the trail straddles the very edge of Black Creek, often in bottomland forests, before climbing up to pine bluffs that give a bird's eye view of the river. Here too, streams cut deep ravines that add vertical variation to the hike. The Black Creek Trail then traverses the longest stretch of pine hill country, passing an old Civilian Conservation Corps campsite, before working its way back to Black Creek, after passing through an open, pine wetland where insect-eating pitcher plants thrive. The final stretch along Black Creek offers one last opportunity to admire the deep woods, scenic waters, and long sandbars before the trail's end at Big Creek Landing.

Overnight camping opportunities are nearly limitless. Water and flat spots are frequent. Many backpackers like to camp on the sandbars for scenery, breezes, and escape from the mosquitoes, which can be

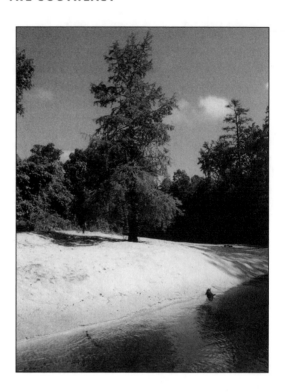

Cypress tree growing
on a sandbar

troublesome in late spring, early summer, and after thunderstorms. However, the shoulder seasons are ideal for trail travel, namely the months of March, April, October, and November, and winter is a viable option. In summer, hot days, warm nights, and annoying insects keep away most sane backpackers. The BCT is moderately used and backpackers seeking solitude will have it any time of year during the week. Weekends won't be bad, and the numerous camping possibilities assure solitude for those willing to find it.

Another upside is a local shuttle service for one-way hikers. Black Creek Canoe Rental not only rents canoes and offers shuttle services for Black Creek paddlers, they also serve hikers and backpackers who want to hike a portion of the trail or tackle it from end to end. I have used their service and highly recommend them.

No instantly accessible resupply points exist along the Black Creek Trail. However, backpackers can easily carry enough food and gear for the 41-mile trip, whether they do it in 3, 4, 5, or 6 nights. Be apprised that at one point, the path does venture about a mile from the hamlet of

Brooklyn, where there are a couple of small stores, selling snacks and such. Black Creek Canoe Rental, also in Brooklyn, has some camp supplies. The only real downside for hikers is Camp Shelby, a nearby military installation that occasionally explodes bombs, breaking the area's solitude. Overall, the Black Creek experience is not one to be missed. For a two-pronged adventure, consider doing what I have done in the past, canoeing a few days down Black Creek, travelling the 31 miles from Big Creek Landing to Fairley Bridge Landing, then backpacking up the Black Creek Trail, 41 miles from Fairley Bridge Landing back to Big Creek Landing.

# Black Creek Trail, Fairley Bridge Landing to Janice Landing

| | |
|---|---|
| **Length:** | 16.6 miles |
| **Trail Condition:** | Excellent |
| **Highs:** | Black Creek Wilderness |
| **Lows:** | Potential mosquito problems |
| **Season:** | Best during early spring, fall, and winter |
| **Difficulty:** | Moderate |
| **Use:** | Moderate |
| **Tips:** | Camp on sandbars if the insects are troublesome |
| **Campsites:** | Numerous |

**FAIRLEY BRIDGE TRAILHEAD:** From the junction of US 49 and MS 26 at Wiggins, head east on MS 26 for 0.9 miles to MS 29. Head north on MS 29 for 7 miles to Fairley Bridge Road. Turn right on Fairley Bridge Road for 6 miles to FR 374. Turn right on FR 374 and follow it 0.1 miles to FR 374A. Turn left on FR 374A and follow it 0.7 miles to end at Fairley Bridge Landing. The Black Creek Trail starts at the rear of the camping area here, near the rest room.

**JANICE TRAILHEAD:** From the junction of US 49 and MS 26 at Wiggins, head east on MS 26 for 0.9 miles to MS 29. Head north on MS 29 for 12.7 miles to the Black Creek trailhead parking on the left side of the road. This parking area is actually a short distance before the Janice Landing.

This section of trail begins its upstream trek in the lower Black Creek valley, traversing the thick woods of South Mississippi. Much of the trail lies within the corridor of the federally designated wild and scenic portion of the river. The path then heads for the hills, literally the Red Hills, making the first of many forays into the surprisingly challenging pine forests lining the watershed. The trail inevitably turns toward the river, only to head away again, entering more hill country, where it begins a long winding trek through the Black Creek Wilderness. Down Mill Creek, up Black Creek, and around Beaverdam Creek—the trail meanders among many forest types before exiting the wilderness at a parking area on MS 29 near Janice Landing.

❉    ❉    ❉

The beginning of your Black Creek hiking adventure starts at Fairley Bridge Landing, a popular take-out for canoeists. Land travelers will begin the trail by heading into the woods away from the boat landing near the campground rest room. The foot-only trail, marked with 2-by-6-inch white blazes, immediately enters a bottomland hardwood forest, goes a few feet, and hits the first of over 80 footbridges that span the streams and wetlands of Black Creek.

Overhead are tall sweetgum, water oak, Southern magnolia, and bay trees. The trail wiggles, staying on high ground with a swamp off to the left and Fairley Bridge Landing access road, FR 374A, to your right. Cross a few boardwalks, bisect FR 374A, then come to FR 374. Turn right on FR 374 and span Bug Branch on the road bridge. Keep on the gravel road to reach blacktopped Fairley Bridge Road at 1.0 mile. Cross the road and re-enter woods of pine and yaupon. Yaupon is a brushy understory tree with stiff branches and small leaves. Creek Indians and several other tribes steeped its leaves to make a strong, tea-like beverage, known as the "black drink" by European settlers. Consumed daily as well as during special ceremonies, the drink was high in caffeine and was believed to purify the body and soul.

Keep northwest along the margin of dry woods to your left and wet-lands to your right. A few boardwalks—usually two, parallel, raised planks placed lengthwise—span swampy areas. Red maples grow near these wet locales. Climb in and out of bottoms, spanning intermittent streams on footbridges in the low spots. The footbridges, which stand over deeper drops, are wider and more sturdily built than the boardwalks. Beyond the footbridges, pass through a gas line clearing at mile 1.9.

The trail periodically climbs up short, steep inclines, leaving behind desiccated hollows to enter hickory-oak hills. Keep an eye out for big-leaf magnolias as the trail dips back into hollows. This small tree has 20 to 30 inch leaves that fan out in a circle, looking almost like an umbrella. The path remains evident, occasionally passing over the faint traces of four-wheel drive tracks and old logging roads. At mile 2.5, cross FR 318B-1, which leads right to the Red Hill Cemetery. Keep north on a jeep track and reach a clearing. The jeep track leaves left while the Black Creek Trail turns right as a footpath. Cruise along a narrow ridgeline before dipping down into a lush ravine to span a clear, sand-bottomed stream at mile 2.9. Climb steps and undulate steeply among heavily wooded mini-gorges cutting through the Red Hills. Wind along a curvy narrow ridgeline to reach bottomlands, where there are footbridges, before coming to Black Creek at mile 4.3. Cruise upstream along the swift, coffee-colored waters, stained from vegetational decay, that contrast greatly with sun-bleached streamside sandbars. Parallel an old roadbed beneath mixed woods and pass over a small footbridge. Beyond the footbridge, look right for a side trail leading to a sandbar suitable for camping or picnicking. Pass under a gas line and through a clearing at mile 4.9, to cross a stream on a wide, sturdy footbridge. There are occasional cane patches around. Abruptly turn away from Black Creek, leisurely climbing a stream valley through pine woods, to cross the gas line again at mile 5.7.

The BCT is now in a drier pine-oak-yaupon forest, but does cross footbridges over wet areas. You may hear or see armadillos rooting beneath leaves near the trail, which has taken a westerly tack, working around a private inholding near Black Creek. Continue up the now dry valley in piney woods, switchbacking to reach FR 382-B at mile 6.8. The trail shortly turns northward and climbs to nearly 250 feet in elevation, lofty ground by South Mississippi standards. Cross the gas pipeline again before entering the Black Creek Wilderness. Pass a trailside kiosk, then descend into the Mill Creek drainage on an old roadbed. The woods are mostly pine here, mixed with some sizable holly and dogwood trees. Tulip trees increase in number as the trail traverses a wet-weather margin overlain with concrete. Mill Creek briefly becomes visible and audible as the wide sandy track stays on higher ground then suddenly drops to span Mill Creek on a footbridge at mile 8.6.

Soon, cross a much smaller stream on a footbridge before reaching Black Creek. Wind upstream, sometimes near Black Creek, sometimes not, occasionally bisecting several small streams on footbridges, then pass alongside a wooded, wet swamp. Black gum trees, with their buttressed bases, emerge from the water, along with cypress trees. At mile 10.1, cross Black Branch on a footbridge. Much cane grows in the bottoms here. Step over more boardwalks before nearing Black Creek in rich, shady woods, where the trail is lined with bay trees. At mile 10.9, a faint trail leads down to Black Creek. Across the water is a huge curved sandbar, the only major bar for a long piece and a nice place to take a break or camp. You have to ford Black Creek to reach it, so if you choose to ford here, do so downstream of the bar. Otherwise, keep forward on the BCT and cross a few slow-moving branches on footbridges in sun dappled woodland. Cross a fourth bridge near an oxbow swamp pond, with ultradark-stained waters. At mile 11.5, a small side path leads right, to the swamp pond, where magnolias grow tall along the water's edge. The trail keeps taking the only high ground around, with wetter margins on both sides before it comes directly alongside Black Creek, with good water views. Keep a sharp eye peeled here, as the trail makes an acute left turn, up incoming Beaverdam Creek; confusing side trails lead forward to camping areas at the confluence of Beaverdam Creek and Black Creek. Continuing on the trail, Beaverdam Creek is now to your right. Notice the occasional palmetto here. Most of the trunk of this palm grows underground, and only the green pointed fan shaped leaves show. In times past, the leaves of this tree were used to make hats and baskets, among other things.

Dip in and out of small bottoms, rising to more open pine woods. At mile 13.0, bridge a small, perennial feeder branch of Beaverdam Creek. Pick up a ridgeline and begin climbing in pineland mixed with yaupon. Atop a hill, at mile 13.8, a side trail leads left to Andrews Chapel. Older, taller pines now predominate. Descend to reach MS 29 at mile 14.2. Turn right along the road, crossing Beaverdam Creek on the road bridge, and keep forward for 0.1 miles. Look right for a foot trail, marked with signs, leading back into the woods. Drop off the roadbed and now work your way back downstream along Beaverdam Creek. Briefly come alongside Beaverdam Creek at mile 14.7, then pass by a slough with still, dark waters. Span some footbridges, dipping in and out of wet areas to reach Beaverdam Creek one more time at mile 15.9. Turn northwest, picking up an old woods road that makes for easy forest travel. Span one last slow branch, and pass a trailside kiosk just before coming to MS 29 just south of the Janice boat landing. Cross the blacktop road and come to a parking area at mile 16.6 and the end of this section. It is 24.1 miles farther to the trail terminus at Big Creek Landing.

# Black Creek Trail, Janice Landing to Big Creek Landing

| | |
|---|---|
| **Length:** | 24.1 miles |
| **Trail Condition:** | Good to excellent |
| **Highs:** | Rich wetlands, streamside environment, pitcher plants |
| **Lows:** | Poorly marked trail in places |
| **Season:** | Best during early spring, fall, and winter |
| **Difficulty:** | Moderate |
| **Use:** | Moderate |
| **Tips:** | Safer parking is at Black Creek Canoe Rental in Brooklyn, rather than Big Creek Landing |

**JANICE LANDING TRAILHEAD:** From the junction of US 49 and MS 26 at Wiggins, head east on MS 26 for 0.9 miles to MS 29. Head north on MS 29 for 12.7 miles to the Black Creek trailhead parking on the left side of the road. This parking area is actually a short distance before the Janice Landing.

**BIG CREEK LANDING TRAILHEAD:** From the junction of US 49 and US 98 on the south side of Hattiesburg, drive south on US 49 for

14.4 miles to Carnes Road. Turn right on Carnes Road and follow it for 0.5 miles to CR 335, Rock Hill-to-Brooklyn Road. Turn right on Rock Hill-to-Brooklyn Road and follow it 3.7 miles to FR 335. Turn right on FR 335 and follow it for just a short distance to FR 335E and follow it for 0.7 miles to a dead end at Big Creek Landing. The trailhead is on the downstream side of the landing.

This section of the BCT stays along its namesake stream more than the lower section, making for easier access to the cool waters and those white sandbars. It is also harder to follow in spots, so have your eyes peeled for those white blazes. Leave the parking area near Janice and soon come to Black Creek, keeping along the stream before meandering in thick woods to reach a segment of bottomland replete with numerous swamps, sloughs, and wetlands. Work your way into pine country, where the open wetlands host many insect-eating pitcher plants. Return streamside near Moodys Landing, where the trail follows Black Creek for several miles, nearing sandbars and climbing to piney bluffs offering great river views. Head into hill country again, where longleaf pines grow tall near the site of an old, abandoned Civilian Conservation Corps camp. Cross busy US 49, then make your most extensive pine-land walk before returning to Black Creek and its lush bottomland hardwoods. The last few miles of the trek stay streamside until the path arrives at Big Creek Landing and its northern terminus.

❂    ❂    ❂

The Black Creek Trail leaves the MS 29 parking area on the opposite end of the parking area from the General Jackson Interpretive Trail, a 0.2-mile-long path, which connects to the Black Creek Trail. It tells of Andrew Jackson's journey from Mobile to New Orleans en route to fight the British during the War of 1812. Jackson and his troops, many of them Tennesseans, crossed Black Creek near here. You can start this section by walking the interpretive trail and intersecting the BCT, or following the BCT as it leaves the parking area near a trail signboard, passing under a power line to soon meet the General Jackson Interpretive Trail. Continue forward to reach a boardwalk then a gravel road. Turn right at the gravel road, which soon forks, and look for the trail heading into the woods between the forks. Bridge a small wetland at 0.5 miles, and soon cross another gravel road to come alongside Black Creek. The creek is much smaller here than when it was last seen many miles downstream. Briefly walk along a forest road and return to the creek. Drop down to a gum swamp among big trees. Cross a perennial stream into a swampy area.

Eventually, turn away from the creek onto high ground at mile 1.9. Pass an area where the forest has been thinned. The trail moves away from the forest and stays mostly level. At mile 2.5, traverse a long boardwalk that leads to a footbridge over a sluggish stream the color of strong coffee. This area has many old woods roads that can be deceiving, so watch for the white blazes. At mile 3.7, return to Black Creek on a bluff. Stay alongside the waterway, bridging a 12-foot deep ravine through which a clear stream flows. The trail begins a pattern of moving toward, then turning away from the river, as it circumvents a slough or rough terrain, sometimes spanning streams or dry ravines along the way. At mile 6.3, the trail enters a mostly dry swampbed, snaking amid widely buttressed gum and cypress trees. Climb just a bit to enter a shady grove of tall magnolia trees. Keep forward here, as an old woods road leaves left and another trail leads right, down to a sandbar. Past this point, the Black Creek Trail tries to straddle dry terrain between wetlands on one side and Black Creek on the other. Just a few feet in elevation changes the forest types here. Look for mountain laurel, with its pinkish-white April blooms, alongside the trail. This small tree or bush has reddish bark and waxy green leaves.

Eventually, climb into hill country, passing many footbridges and boardwalks as you steadily gain elevation. Enter hill country in earnest at mile 7.5, climbing a steep hill straight up a ridgeline. Soon, drop down to a swift sand-bottomed stream at mile 7.7. Bridge the stream to climb another piney hill that shows evidence of burning years back. Step onto a boardwalk of perhaps 100 yards in length. Look for pitcher plants in the open grasses alongside the planks. These carnivorous plants trap insects then consume them. Stay in open pine woods to reach FR 319G at mile 8.4. Dive back down into rich woods and pick up another boardwalk and bridge in a lush, fern-laden wetland. Begin a pattern of climbing in pinelands and dropping down to clear streams. Watch out for faint woods roads distracting from the true trail. The forest transitions to hardwoods as the trail crosses one last clear stream on a footbridge before reaching ever-diminishing-in-size Black Creek at mile 9.8.

Head upstream through woods rich with magnolia, beech, and water oak. For several miles, the glistening waters and shimmering sandbars of Black Creek are nearby. In the short term, keep an eye out across the stream, where a large sandbar and small parking area indicate Moodys Landing at mile 10.1. This landing and camping area can be used as an emergency exit point. The trail dips down and goes right along the river near the upper end of this sandbar, which offers the best opportunity for fording if necessary. In places, the path may be washed out from floods or overgrown among the lush streamside vegetation. There may also be fallen trees. Watch for deer feeding in the area, too. Sandbars on both sides of the river are plentiful and accessible, for those so inclined.

Continuing on, bridge several streams and pass four-wheel drive tracks before climbing to a piney riverside blufftop overlooking Black Creek at mile 12.3. Stay on the bluff, with good views as it alternately becomes cut with steep, wet ravines through which the trail dips then rises back to the bluff. The bluff gives way to hardwoods as the Black Creek Trail crosses one last footbridge over a sandy stream at mile 13.9. Turn abruptly left (southwest) to moderately ascend along the stream, eventually turning away from the unnamed watercourse to reach FR 319F-1 at mile 14.2. Turn right on FR 319F-1, passing a residence. Reach blacktop FR 319F at mile 31.3 and turn right. Follow the road just a short distance, then look left for the foot trail leading back into the woods. Slowly ascend in piney woods, topping a rise to bridge an intermittent streambed, then reach a boardwalk and small bridge over a clear stream that provides the last good water for a while. Just past this, at mile 32.1, approach paved CR 308-E. Cross the paved road and walk a couple of very long and snake-like boardwalks, the most curvy ones on the entire trail. Notice how even the pines in this part-time wetland have buttressed bases to keep upright during wet periods. Keep a westward track, ascending to an unnumbered forest road at mile 33.3, topping out at nearly 270 feet in elevation, the highest of the entire trail.

Work southeast through rolling pine woods to reach CR 316, at mile 17.6. Look left here, and walk the blacktop briefly, before dropping back into a longleaf pine woodland on the far side of the road. Keep south on an old woods road and look for the young sprouts of longleaf pines on the trailside. These young trees grow upward with no limbs for several years, using their energy to rise above low level fires that often creep through

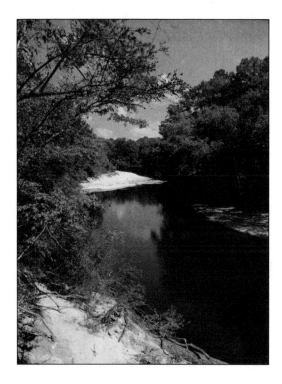

Bluff view of Black Creek

this forest type. The trail turns right and soon enters the cleared parking area, near the site of the old CCC camp from the 1930s. The trail follows old pine needle–carpeted woods roads westward to reach the Illinois Central Gulf Railroad at mile 18.3. Walk a few steps left along the tracks, then look for a trail on the far side of the tracks that dips over a small bridge and climbs a few steps to reach busy US 49.

Cross the divided highway heading toward the gravel Boyt Road. The Black Creek Trail re-enters the woods just to the right of the gravel road. Turn away from the highway in lush woods, crossing a short bridge over an intermittent streambed, then climb into pines to reach FR 348 at mile 18.8. Turn right and follow FR 348 as it dips down, then rises to a hilltop. Pay close attention here, as the trail re-enters the woods to the right just as the road makes a sharp left near a "Children At Play" sign. Veer right into the forest on a grassy woods lane. After around 75 yards, the grassy lane forks. Veer left and descend to reach a long boardwalk and footbridge spanning Macklin Creek at mile 19.6.

Resume the boardwalk beyond the bridge and climb away, curving northward to cross CR 334 at mile 19.8. The BCT is marked with white plastic diamonds at this point; in the future it may be marked with these diamonds elsewhere on the trail. Stay primarily in pine woods, occasionally dipping into moister margins with footbridges to reach a distinct woods road in longleaf pines. Veer right on the needle-carpeted road that thins out into a footpath and drops a few more times before reaching CR 341 at mile 21.3. Keep forward, dipping a bit to reach blacktop CR 335 at mile 21.4. Veer left across the road. The BCT angles up to reach a small knob, then dips down to swampland, which the trail hasn't seen in a while. Cross this wetland on a boardwalk. You are now back in the rich bottomland forest of the Black Creek floodplain. Drop down again, then span a footbridge at the confluence of two small branches to once again reach Black Creek at mile 21.9.

A quick break in a power-line clearing is the only change in the lush forest. Keep directly along Black Creek, rollercoastering down to cross feeder streams on footbridges, then climbing once again. River views and sandbar access points are numerous. Pines tower over the junglesque scenery. At mile 22.6, the trail passes by two small cabins. The trail turns away from the river here and works around the private property, then crosses the cabin access road to re-enter full blown woodland. Soon descend to a wide, sturdy footbridge with handrails over Granny Creek at mile 22.9. Pick up an old woods road and meander along Black Creek, resuming a course through bottomland broken by wet and dry ravines. Some are bridged, some are not. Grab a few final river views just before arriving at Big Creek Landing and the northwest terminus of the Black Creek Trail at mile 24.1. Here is a picnic area, canoe launch, and trailhead parking area, though I recommend using Black Creek Canoe Rental in nearby Brooklyn for safer parking and shuttle service.

## Black Creek Trail Log

### FAIRLEY BRIDGE LANDING TO JANICE LANDING

| | | |
|---|---|---|
| 0.0 | 40.7 | Leave Fairley Bridge Landing and enter woods, curving north |
| 1.0 | 39.7 | Cross black-topped Fairley Bridge Road, enter pine woods, dropping down to wet margins |

## Black Creek Trail Log *(continued)*

| | | |
|---|---|---|
| **1.9** | **38.8** | Pass through gas line clearing. Big-leaved magnolias prevalent beyond forest road |
| **2.5** | **38.2** | Cross FR 318B-1, briefly keep north on old jeep track, then veer right on footpath |
| **2.9** | **37.8** | Bridge clear sand-bottomed stream, undulate through Red Hills |
| **4.3** | **36.4** | Come alongside Black Creek, sandbars are accessible via side trails |
| **4.9** | **35.8** | Pass through gas line clearing, cross stream on wide footbridge |
| **5.7** | **35.0** | Pass gas line clearing again, after abruptly turning away from Black Creek |
| **6.8** | **33.9** | Enter Black Creek Wilderness, take wide sandy track in burned woods |
| **8.6** | **32.1** | Span noisy Mill Creek on footbridge, soon reach Black Creek in bottomland hardwoods |
| **10.1** | **30.6** | Span Black Branch on footbridge in swampy cane bottom |
| **10.9** | **29.8** | Faint trail leads down to Black Creek to access huge curved sandbar across stream |
| **11.5** | **29.2** | Come alongside swamp ponds, then make acute left turn, now heading upstream along Beaverdam Creek. |
| **13.0** | **27.7** | Span feeder branch of Beaverdam Creek on footbridge, ascend into pine woods. |
| **13.8** | **26.9** | Side trail leads left to Andrews Chapel |
| **14.2** | **26.5** | Reach MS 29. Turn right and span Beaverdam Creek on road bridge |
| **14.3** | **26.4** | Re-enter woods on foot trail leading right |
| **14.7** | **26.0** | Come alongside Beaverdam Creek at confluence with feeder branch |
| **15.9** | **24.8** | Come alongside Beaverdam Creek again, then turn away on old woods road |
| **16.6** | **24.1** | Cross blacktopped MS 29 and come to trail parking near Janice Landing |

## JANICE LANDING TO BIG CREEK LANDING

| | | |
|---|---|---|
| **17.1** | **23.6** | Span wetland on footbridge, soon come alongside Black Creek in swampy bottomland |
| **19.1** | **21.6** | Traverse long boardwalk far from Black Creek over dark stream |
| **20.3** | **20.4** | Return to Black Creek, now on a bluff, keep generally near river |
| **22.9** | **17.8** | Reach magnolia grove. Side trail leads right, down to sandbar on river. Black Creek Trail continues forward in wet areas on many footbridges. |
| **24.3** | **16.4** | Reach long boardwalk through pine country. Look for pitcher plants |

## Black Creek Trail Log *(continued)*

| | | |
|---|---|---|
| **25.0** | **15.7** | Cross FR 319G |
| **26.4** | **14.3** | Come alongside ever-diminishing Black Creek, head upstream for long distance |
| **26.7** | **14.0** | Emergency exit point at Moodys Landing across river. Undulate along river |
| **28.9** | **11.8** | Piney bluff offers good river view. Dip in and out of ravines cutting through bluff |
| **30.5** | **10.2** | Turn left ascending alongside feeder stream |
| **30.8** | **9.9** | Reach and cross FR 319F-1. Turn right and follow road |
| **31.3** | **9.4** | Reach and follow blacktopped FR 319F right short distance |
| **31.4** | **9.3** | Turn left from 319F onto foot trail entering woods |
| **32.1** | **8.6** | Cross paved CR 308E. Keep in low, wet woods with long boardwalks |
| **33.3** | **7.4** | Cross non-numbered forest road near top of hill, 270 feet high |
| **34.2** | **6.5** | Cross CR 316. |
| **34.9** | **5.8** | Reach US 49, after passing by old CCC camp and crossing Illinois Central Gulf Railroad, re-enter woods |
| **35.4** | **5.3** | Emerge onto FR 348. Turn right on gravel road |
| **36.2** | **4.5** | Cross Macklin Creek on footbridge |
| **36.4** | **4.3** | Cross CR 334, stay in pine woods |
| **37.9** | **2.8** | Cross CR 341 |
| **38.0** | **2.7** | Cross CR 335, drop back down to Black Creek in bottomland |
| **38.5** | **2.2** | Reach Black Creek, many sandbars and river access points |
| **39.2** | **1.5** | Swing around two small cabin inholdings |
| **39.5** | **1.2** | Span Granny Creek on sturdy footbridge. Meander along Black Creek |
| **40.7** | **0.0** | Big Creek Landing, end of trail |

## Black Creek Trail Information

De Soto National Forest
654 Frontage Road
P.O. Box 248
Wiggins, Mississippi 39577
(601) 928-5291
www.fs.fed.us/r8/miss

Black Creek Canoe Rental
P.O. Box 414
Brooklyn, Mississippi 39425
(601) 582-8884
www.blackcreekcanoe.com

# FLORIDA TRAIL

Hiking in Florida is a little known and underrated outdoor recreation opportunity. The development and evolution of the master path of the state, the Florida National Scenic Trail, is bringing attention to the quality hiking found throughout this southern land. A long hiking season is ideal for walking during times when weather can be unpleasant elsewhere.

There is more to the landscape than appears at first glance. Most would describe the terrain here as flat. However, in Florida small changes in elevation make big differences. A few feet can result in wildly different habitats, as surely as thousands of feet change habitats in the Rocky Mountains. A small hill in Florida may harbor pine woods, then a nearly imperceptible depression leads to a lush subtropical swamp.

Water is a major element of most Florida hiking experiences, whether it is walking through a subtropical swamp, hiking alongside a spring-fed pond, or crossing a blackwater creek. Building the Florida Trail has been a long and massive undertaking, with much work left to be done. To do the entire FT requires much road walking at the present time. From the FT I have gleaned three complete foot-trail-only sections that traverse federal lands in the state and make for great multinight experiences in the real, natural Florida.

The first section makes a 41-mile traverse of the Big Cypress National Preserve. Located in the heart of South Florida, this marks the beginning of the entire FT and traverses through cypress swamps, pine islands, and open sawgrass prairies amid 700,000 acres of wild land. The second section showcases another Florida environment, sand pine scrub forest—a unique habitat, the largest remaining tract of which is found along the 60-mile course of FT in the Ocala National Forest. The third section offers a mosaic of different environments along its 67 miles—hardwood swamps, longleaf pine/wiregrass ecosystems, titi thickets, and open savannas in the Apalachicola National Forest.

# *Florida Trail,*
# *Big Cypress National Preserve*

The Big Cypress National Preserve adjoins the north side of the Everglades National Park, covering over 700,000 acres of cypress sloughs, pinelands, tropical hammocks, and freshwater marshes. The entire FT starts its northward journey here, and it starts off with a bang. The trail here is rough, rugged, and remote, while passing through some incredible scenery. Have you ever walked through a dwarf cypress swamp? The FT leaves Loop Road and wastes no time in initiating hikers into "swamp slogging" through picturesque cypress sloughs, crossing Roberts Lakes Strand, where water far outweighs dry land, eventually reaching the Tamiami Trail, at US 41.

The FT continues north beyond the Tamiami Trail. Wet feet are the norm here, too. Hikers must also contend with crossing muddy swamp buggy roads. But this inconvenience is well worth the views. It's not all watery though; cypress soughs often give way to pine islands and prairies, offering continually changing landscapes. These pine islands allow camping and are also habitat for deer. And where there are deer, there is the Florida panther—deer is its preferred fare. The panther needs remoteness, too, and the Big Cypress has plenty of that, especially farther north on the FT. Tree islands become more lush, with palms and eventually tropical trees, such as gumbo limbo and Simpson stopper. In the extreme north of the preserve, cypress trees once again dominate, and the tree islands act as dry waysides for resting and camping.

During the 1800s, it was in the expanse that is now the Big Cypress where the Seminoles hid, outfoxing U.S. troops until the federals gave up searching for the wiley American natives. Backpackers will find that the trip on the FT from Loop Road to I-75 is one of the most unique trips ever, and will understand why the Seminoles chose the Big Cypress to make their last stand.

# Big Cypress National Preserve, Loop Road to Tamiami Trail

| | |
|---|---|
| **Length:** | 9.3 miles |
| **Trail Condition:** | Fair to poor |
| **Highs:** | Cypress swamps, isolation |
| **Lows:** | Completely submerged path, irregular limestone footing, poorly marked trail |
| **Season:** | Winter and very early spring |
| **Difficulty:** | Potentially strenuous walking through water |
| **Use:** | Moderate to low |
| **Tips:** | Have boots suited for wet conditions, consider using trekking poles |
| **Campsites:** | 2.4 and 3.5 miles |

**LOOP ROAD TRAILHEAD:** From the Oasis Visitor Center at Big Cypress National Preserve, take US 41, Tamiami Trail, east for 14.8 miles to Loop Road. Turn right on Loop Road and follow it for 13.5 miles to the FT, which starts on your right. Look for a stripe painted across Loop Road marking the trail.

**TAMIAMI TRAIL TRAILHEAD:** This section of the FT starts at the Oasis Visitor Center at Big Cypress National Preserve on US 41, 21 miles east the junction of US 41 and Collier CR 29 in Everglades City.

This is the wettest and most unusual section of long trail in the Southeast. The FT leaves Loop Road, the southern terminus of the entire FT, and heads north through a nearly continuous bald cypress woodland that is underwater most of the year, including the drier winter hiking season. Even in the best of times it may be inundated 50% of its distance, but more likely around 95%. Prepare for wet feet on the entire trail and possibly water to your knees at times. Before hiking this section of the FT, call Big Cypress Preserve to check on water levels.

All this wetness may seem daunting. On the other hand, it demystifies swamps to a degree: you will be hiking through one. The path also meanders through sawgrass prairies, by tree islands, and through Robert Lakes Strand, where the towering cypresses covered in air plants and ferns, tropical hammocks, and clear flowing water offer a wild Florida landscape. Dry campsites can normally be found at 2.4 and 3.5 miles.

❋   ❋   ❋

Start this section by heading north from Loop Road and immediately drop into a bald cypress forest that will most likely be wet. The water below is clear and harbors much aquatic life. The cypress trees soon grow tall. Pocked limestone makes for irregular footing—watch your step. Occasional slash pines are on higher spots. Keep an eye peeled for the orange blazes, as animal paths sometimes cross the wet FT.

At mile 1.2, pass a small tree island on the right, then enter a sawgrass prairie with scattered small cypress. At mile 2.1, pass a pine island before coming to a larger pine-palm hammock on trail-right at mile 2.4. This one usually has dry ground and potential camping or sitting spots. Return to open prairie, which melds into cypress woods with an understory of sawgrass. Pines stay to the east with occasional tree islands scattered among the cypress.

Emerge into a pine-palm hammock at mile 3.5. A campsite stands atop high ground on trail-left with a fire ring and a pump well for water. Leave the hammock and re-enter a sawgrass prairie. Once again cypress trees slowly increase in size and number. This increase peaks out in a tall cypress stand. Watch for a sharp right turn in the center of the stand. Leave the bald cypress and follow the path as it "climbs" to higher ground and a full-blown hardwood hammock, heavy with ferns at mile 5.5.

Abruptly drop down into a cypress swamp. The trail is now crossing the Roberts Lakes Strand. Here, clumps of dry soil, rich with vegetation, alternate with clear moving water from which widely buttressed cypresses emerge. Keep an eye on the blazes here, as the trail unexpectedly veers left and begins to follow an old logging tram road due west at mile 5.9.

Stay with the old tram road alongside cypress trees until mile 6.5, where the westward course abruptly turns north, to the right, still in medium-size cypress. The trail is poorly marked here. At mile 7.9, the cypress woods thicken and the water correspondingly deepens. The FT is now in the middle of a cypress dome, an area where the trees stand taller than others on the horizon and resemble a dome. Trees decrease in size until entering another cypress dome at mile 8.5. The trailside woods gradually thin out to a sawgrass prairie before reaching Tamiami Trail and the Oasis Visitor Center at mile 9.3. The FT continues across Tamiami Trail (US 41), crossing the northern Big Cypress Preserve, and ending at I-75 in 32 miles.

# Big Cypress National Preserve, Tamiami Trail to I-75

| | |
|---|---|
| **Length:** | 32.0 miles |
| **Trail Condition:** | Fair to very poor |
| **Highs:** | Cypress sloughs, pine islands, wildlife, isolation, navigational challenge |
| **Lows:** | Poorly marked trail, wet hiking, navigational challenge |
| **Season:** | Winter and very early spring |
| **Difficulty:** | Depends on water level, can be difficult if water is up |
| **Use:** | Low |
| **Tips:** | If you are unskilled at route finding, consider using a GPS; stay with the orange blazes, immediately backtracking if losing them |
| **Campsites:** | 7.2, 10.1, 17.8, and 24.1 miles |

**TAMIAMI TRAIL TRAILHEAD:** This section of the FT starts at the Oasis Visitor Center at Big Cypress National Preserve on US 41, 21 miles east of Everglades City from the junction of US 41 and Collier CR 29.

**I-75 TRAILHEAD:** This trailhead is located at the major rest stop about 35 miles east from the beginning of the toll portion of I-75 near Naples.

This section of the FT traverses some of the most rugged terrain in Florida, the Big Cypress National Preserve. The hiking will be challenging; wet feet and slogging through water up to your knees are guaranteed. The sun can be brutal in open areas. And following the orange blazes of the often-faint trail takes a keen eye and patience.

The "Big" in Big Cypress refers to the size of the 700,000-acre swamp, not the size of the trees, and after this walk you will understand the meaning of the word. The trail is characterized by miles and miles of poorly marked cypress sloughs, punctuated by slash pine–sabal palm hammocks and rich, tropical hardwood hammocks. Adequately spaced campsites and ample water along the way make the "Big Cype" a

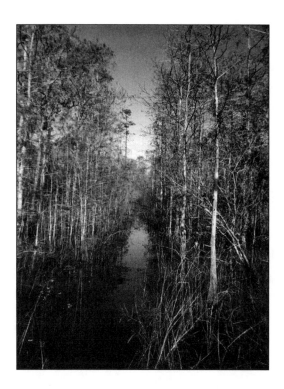

The Florida Trail's
portentous beginning

backpacker's paradise. Normally, backpackers are looking for water to go with some level ground. Here, backpackers are looking for dry ground to go along with their water. Campsites are normally found at 7.2, 10.1, 17.8, and 24.1 miles along the trail. A hike through the Big Cypress will help you understand why this area is one of the last strongholds of the Florida panther. Be prepared for serious backcountry hiking when entering the Big Cypress.

Some folks who get back here drive "swamp buggies." These contraptions look like Jeeps on steroids, with their oversized tires and elevated frames. They make wide muddy paths, which the FT crosses. But traversing the Big Cypress via foot power will give you a unique experience, which is simply unlike hiking anywhere else in the United States.

Begin this section of the FT by departing from the west end of the Oasis Visitor Center and following the orange-blazed trail between two fences and along a canal. Soon turn right, still following the fence line on an elevated roadbed that borders an airstrip. Begin heading north, the primary direction for the hike. A sawgrass prairie extends to the west.

At 0.4 miles, make the first of several swamp buggy trail crossings. Palm and cypress trees border the trail. Reach the first pine island at mile 1.0. The path is drier here. Overhead grow tall slash pines, shade palms, and palmettos. Occasional hardwood hammocks are scattered among the evergreens.

Watch your footing over the mud and pocked limestone as cypress trees become more prevalent. Watch also for the markings of the FT, which can be standard orange blazes on trees or orange flagging tape tied around trees. The trail begins to alternate between drier pine-palm hammocks and wet cypress-sawgrass complexes.

At mile 3.0, after a glut of swamp buggy trails, come to the blue-blazed Blue Loop, leaving left. This side trail is very poorly and sporadically maintained and not at all recommended, though it will be restored and re-blazed in the future. Stay forward on the FT, as it keeps north through increasing palms and hardwoods. At mile 3.8, traverse a very muddy area of swamp buggy roads, then pass through a wet cypress slough at mile 4.2. The trail mainly stays in pine-palm-palmetto areas connected by cypress.

At mile 6.0, the trail steps over limestone pocked with particularly deep holes, often filled with water. The FT opens onto a cypress slough, then emerges into pineland, where exotic melaleuca trees grow. These invaders are identified by their paper-like white bark and tall, narrow profile. Originally from Australia, melaleucas were brought to Florida as border-forming ornamental trees. Since melaleucas trees prefer wet or moist areas, the Big Cypress habitat unfortunately proved to be an all too perfect environment for them. This tree is also the subject of an urban legend. Maybe you have heard it: Melaleuca trees are so widespread because a greedy land speculator spread their seeds by airplane in order to dry and then develop the many wetlands in South Florida. No matter the origin, melaleucas are considered one of the Sunshine State's worst invaders, being nearly impossible to eradicate.

At mile 7.2, just to the right of the trail in a pine-palm-palmetto area, is Seven Mile Camp. The camp is shaded by wax myrtle. A fire ring, sitting logs, a pocked limestone hole filled with water, and an old capped well mark the camp. Keep north past Seven Mile Camp, and at 7.4 miles pass the blue-blazed westward shortcut to the Blue Loop. This neglected shortcut is not recommended, although it is slated for future mainte-nance. The footbed of the FT becomes more faint beyond the Seven Mile Camp area—keep your eyes on the orange blazes as you pass through mixed pine and cypress areas. Many of the cypress trees are below head level and crowd the trail. The vegetation in this flat land changes with the slightest variation in elevation.

At mile 10.1, come to an exceptionally large and wide pine island. The slash pines overhead are noticeably tall. Soon come to a pile of lime-stone rocks on the trail. This is Ten Mile Camp and is much less used than Seven Mile Camp. You will have to get water from cypress domes here. Continue northeast and once again dive into the cypress. Keep alternating between cypress and pine until you enter an extended cypress strand at mile 11.6, now heading northwest. Before, predominate pinelands were bridged by cypress sloughs. Now, predominate cypress sloughs are bridged by sporadic pinelands.

At mile 12.4, the trail circles around an immense prairie of head-high sawgrass to your left. Leave the tall sawgrass and head through a mixed landscape of prairies, cypress woods, and pine islands. At mile

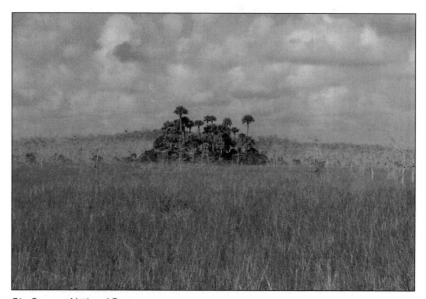

Big Cypress National Preserve

15.0, reach the northern terminus of the blue-blazed Blue Loop. This end of the Blue Loop is even more remote and poorly marked than the previous junctions and may very well be missed by most hikers. Look for the loop where the FT turns sharply right here, to the north, heading into open pine woods.

Follow the orange blazes through pine islands, cypress sloughs, and sawgrass prairies. Palms become more prevalent as you enter drier lands. Briefly pass through tall, thick sawgrass near palm trees at mile 16.5. Keep a constant watch for the orange blazes. At mile 17.8, enter the hammock of Thirteen Mile Camp. Even from a distance, this tree island is clearly more lush than those previously passed. Once in here, there is a profusion of cabbage palms and hardwood hammock species such as live oak. The sure sign you are at Thirteen Mile Camp is the broken hand-pump well in the hammock's center. This is an excellent campsite.

The FT continues north out of Thirteen Mile Camp, crossing a swamp buggy road to enter a cypress slough. Soon, start a pattern of walking through sloughs and crossing palm-pine lands. Though the trail makes many twists and turns, it generally keeps a northward course. More abrupt turns are marked with double orange blazes. At mile 19.3, pass a prairie dotted with sawn stumps of cypress and pine. Soon, bypass two bamboo stands in succession. Simply put, the trail is hard to follow here. As soon as you lose the trail, immediately backtrack to the last blaze or flagging tape you saw, then re-orient until you find the next blaze. Do not continue if you stop finding blazes.

Cypress woods become more dominant, with numerous tall domes on the horizon. At mile 21.1, the FT reaches a barbed wire fence to the left. Walk alongside the fence for 0.2 miles, then head north, away from the fence. At mile 21.9, the FT makes an abrupt left turn off a swamp buggy road it has picked up. Enter a pine-palm hammock but soon slog through more sloughs. Come alongside a rich tropical hammock on your left at mile 22.3. Live oak, ferns, coco plum, and other plants make a shady, dry resting spot. Soon, pass two more rich hammocks.

Continue north through a sea of cypress dotted with small tree islands. The swamp deepens before coming to a large, especially rich tropical hammock on the right at mile 24.1. This hammock has very tall live oak, palms, gumbo limbo, Simpson stoppers, and other lush vegetation. In times past, a path was cut to the center of the hammock, where a campsite lies. The year-round growing season can quickly obliterate camps, but this hammock has been a traditional camping spot and has remained intact.

Beyond this hammock the FT enters a deeper swamp again, where you can expect water to your knees or higher. Pass smaller tree islands on the horizon. Keep north, then northwest through mostly cypress for quite a distance, though the pine-palm and sawgrass prairies ecosystems are represented. At mile 28.3, cross three swamp buggy roads in quick succession, the second of which is the primary swamp buggy path to I-75. The FT is now on the west side of this road. Keep slogging through cypress of differing size, shapes, and forms, with bigger cypress indicating deeper water.

By mile 29.1, palm islands appear on a sawgrass horizon. Step onto dry ground at mile 29.3. Enjoy dry footing, if only for a short distance, then make an abrupt right turn to the east and come to the main buggy road connecting to I-75 at mile 29.6. Turn left and follow the wide, muddy trail north before coming to a high metal fence with a gate at mile 31.6. Walk through the gate and turn left, going against the flow of an on-ramp to I-75. Walk 0.4 miles to the I-75 rest area, ending the Big Cypress portion of the FT at mile 32.1. Phones, water, and soft drink machines are located here: quite a change from the wild Big Cypress.

## Florida Trail, Big Cypress Natural Preserve Trail Log

### LOOP ROAD TO TAMIAMI TRAIL

| | | |
|---|---|---|
| 0.0 | 41.8 | FT leaves Loop Road |
| 1.2 | 40.6 | Pass small tree island on right and enter sawgrass prairie |
| 2.1 | 39.7 | Pass pine island |
| 2.4 | 39.4 | Reach pine-palm hammock, dry ground with potential camping |
| 3.5 | 38.3 | Pine-palm hammock, campsite with fire ring, pump well |
| 5.5 | 36.3 | Reach hardwood hammock heavy with ferns, drop down to cypress swamp |
| 5.9 | 35.9 | Follow west-bound tram road after sharp left turn |
| 6.5 | 35.3 | Sharp right turn, FT now heads due north into cypress |
| 7.9 | 33.9 | Cypress woods thicken and water deepens |
| 8.5 | 33.3 | Enter tall cypress dome, woods thin out to become sawgrass prairie |

## Florida Trail, Big Cypress National Preserve Trail Log *(continued)*

| | | |
|---|---|---|
| **9.3** | **32.5** | Reach Tamiami Trail, US 41, and Oasis Visitor Center, cross US 41 and leave west end of visitor center, then turn right, following fence line of airstrip |

### TAMIAMI TRAIL TO I-75

| | | |
|---|---|---|
| **9.7** | **32.1** | Make first of several swamp buggy crossings |
| **10.3** | **31.5** | Reach first pine island, path becomes drier |
| **12.3** | **29.5** | Intersect blue-blazed Blue Loop Trail (not recommended), FT keeps forward |
| **13.1** | **28.7** | Traverse very muddy area of swamp buggy roads |
| **13.5** | **28.3** | Pass through very wet cypress slough |
| **15.3** | **26.5** | Step over limestone pocked with particularly deep holes |
| **16.5** | **25.3** | Reach Seven Mile Camp just to right of trail, fire ring, sitting logs, and capped well |
| **16.7** | **25.1** | Blue-blazed shortcut to Blue Loop (not recommended), FT becomes more faint |
| **19.4** | **22.4** | Reach exceptionally large and wide pine island, piled rocks mark Ten Mile Camp |
| **20.9** | **19.9** | Enter extended cypress strand, now heading northwest |
| **21.7** | **19.1** | Circle around immense prairie of head-high sawgrass |
| **24.3** | **17.5** | Reach poorly marked north end of Blue Loop, FT turns sharply right here |
| **25.8** | **16.0** | Pass through thick, tall sawgrass near palm trees |
| **27.1** | **14.7** | Enter tree hammock and Thirteen Mile Camp, excellent campsite, broken pump well, water can be obtained from nearby cypress domes |
| **28.6** | **13.2** | Pass prairie dotted with sawn stumps, trail becomes very hard to follow |
| **30.4** | **11.4** | FT reaches barbed wire fence on trail-left, parallel fence |
| **31.2** | **10.6** | Trail makes sharp left turn off swamp buggy road trail has picked up |
| **31.6** | **10.2** | Come alongside rich tropical hammock to left, pass more rich hammocks |
| **33.4** | **8.4** | Hammock on right with tall live oaks, palms, and gumbo limbo, campsite in center of hammock, FT enters vast sawgrass-dwarf cypress prairie broken with tree islands |
| **37.6** | **4.2** | Cross three swamp buggy roads in quick succession |
| **38.4** | **3.4** | Palm islands appear on sawgrass horizon |
| **38.6** | **3.2** | Step onto dry ground, soon make abrupt right turn |
| **39.4** | **2.4** | Reach primary swamp buggy road heading toward I-75, turn left on buggy road |

## Florida Trail, Big Cypress National Preserve Trail Log *(continued)*

**41.4**   **1.4**      Reach high metal fence with gate, walk through gate and turn left

**41.8**   **0.0**      Reach I-75 rest area, end of FT through Big Cypress, phones, water, soft drink machines

## Big Cypress National Preserve Trail Information

Florida Trail Association
5415 SW 13th Street
Gainesville, Florida 32608
(800) 343-1882
www.florida-trail.org

Big Cypress National Preserve
H.C.R. 61, Box 110
Ocohopee, Florida 34141
(941) 695-4111
www.nps.gov/bicy

# Florida Trail,
# Ocala National Forest

The Ocala National Forest, located in north central Florida, is a place of contrasts. On one hand, it has the remnant of rolling, sand-pine scrub hills that once covered much of the central state. Sand-pine scrub is a forest type that grows on fast draining sandy soils. This habitat is often surrounded by scrub oaks and other plants that tolerate the dry conditions. Lands like this are easily developed and have all but disappeared in Florida, adding value to this sand-pine scrub forest—the world's largest. Attendant species such as the scrub jay are equally appreciative of this habitat, upon which they are dependent.

On the other hand, Ocala has numerous natural lakes and springs. Shallow lakes, scattered throughout the forest, are watery oases among the drier hills. Grassy prairies, offering far-reaching views, often surround the lakes. The springs of the Ocala are world famous. Juniper Springs and Alexander Springs have clear, alluring waters in a semitropical setting. Recreation areas, with swimming, nature walks, canoeing, and camping, have sprung up around these springs.

Through these beautiful yet contrasting areas runs a 60-mile segment of the FT. The FT connects Clearwater Lake in the south with Lake Ocklawaha in the north. This section passes by many springs and lakes and through the unique sand-pine scrub. Many hikers consider this portion of the FT, once known as the Ocala Trail, as the crown jewel of the entire Florida National Scenic Trail system. An added hiking bonus is the walk through the Juniper Prairie Wilderness, which captures the Ocala at its most primitive. Backpackers can easily end-to-end hike the entire Ocala, but can resupply at Salt Springs if they choose. The FT passes by several national-forest campgrounds in addition to numerous backcountry camping opportunities. Water can be obtained from both natural lakes, a few creeks, and developed campgrounds.

# Ocala National Forest, Clearwater Lake to Juniper Springs

| | |
|---|---|
| **Length:** | 24.7 miles |
| **Trail Condition:** | Good |
| **Highs:** | Numerous forest environments, spring fed creek, ponds, prairies, and lakes |
| **Lows:** | Sonic booms from nearby naval bombing range |
| **Season:** | Late fall to spring |
| **Difficulty:** | Moderate |
| **Use:** | Moderate |
| **Tips:** | Have hat and sunscreen for sunny portions of trail |
| **Campsites:** | 5.2, 9.3, 13.9, 15.3, 17.2 and 24.7 miles |

**CLEARWATER LAKE TRAILHEAD:** From the Seminole Ranger Station in Umatilla, drive north on SR 19 for 1.5 miles to Lake CR 42. Turn right on Lake CR 42, and head east for 6.3 miles to Clearwater Lake Recreation Area. Since parking at the Lake CR 42 trailhead is less than ideal, the Clearwater Lake parking area is recommended for car shuttles. The trailhead starts on the right, 50 yards after the left turn to the recreation area.

**JUNIPER SPRINGS TRAILHEAD:** From Ocala, drive east on SR 40 for 28 miles to Juniper Springs Recreation Area, on your left. The FT starts on the entrance road to the recreation area. Hikers can choose to park their auto inside the recreation area for a fee.

The FT had its beginnings here in the Ocala National Forest. When built in 1966, it was called the Ocala Trail. Some still call the Ocala portion of the FT by its old name. This section of trail starts out a little tame, then passes some prairie and pond environments. Later, it crosses one of the Ocala's few surface streams, then passes through rolling longleaf-pine land to enter the classic sand-pine scrub for which the national forest is known. The FT then passes through some scenic and remote territory of the Ocala National Forest. The route alternates between the open natural lakes and rolling sand hills of the state's Central Ridge. The lake country features far-reaching views and cool waters. The sand-pine scrub forests cover big hills that offer vertical variation little seen in Florida. Oddly enough, some of the most remote territory on this hike borders a naval bombing range. If the planes are dropping bombs, the booms will pierce your ears.

Camping areas with accessible water can be found at 5.2, 9.3, 13.9, 15.3, 17.2, and 24.7 miles.

❀    ❀    ❀

From Clearwater Lake Recreation parking area, head east on the access trail. Enter a longleaf-pine forest, descend into a flat and climb a bit through oak and sand pine to intersect the FT at 0.2 miles. About 0.3 miles to the right is Lake CR 42 and the actual beginning of the FT. Turn left instead and head north on the orange-blazed FT. The trail crosses the Paisley Woods Bicycle Trail a couple of times, as well as a few obscure jeep and ATV trails, but the course of the FT is rarely in doubt. There will be houses visible on private land to the east. At mile 1.8, cross Paisley Road, then descend and roll through open woods of longleaf pine and scrub oak. Needle-covered sand forms the footbed. Watch for trailside cacti. At mile 3.6, pass a large prairie encircling Duck Pond. Leave the north end of the prairie at mile 4.1 and traverse a nearly pure stand of turkey oaks that gives way to open flatwoods. At mile 4.6, the FT passes under a major power line. Stay right and look for an orange blaze entering a palmetto thicket. The trail passes through longleaf pines until descending to a moister area and Glenn Branch at mile 5.2. This creek has cool, clear water, allowing moisture-loving trees such as maple to thrive. Campsites are in the area.

Cross Glenn Branch on a footbridge and emerge onto a pine flatwood featuring pond, slash, and longleaf pines. At mile 5.7, bisect a junglesque palm-maple-oak swamp on a boardwalk. Encounter more boardwalks before coming out on FR 539 at mile 6.2. Enter mixed-pine flatwoods across the road and turn northwest to cross a small prairie to the left at mile 6.5. Soon after this, the forest transitions to sand pine and

its attendant scrub-oak understory. Cross FR 538-E at mile 7.8. As
the trail nears Alexander Springs, the woods drop off sharply toward
the spring run. At mile 8.9, take a long boardwalk over a sporadically
wet area and reach the junction with the Alexander Springs Spur Trail at
mile 9.3.

The Alexander Springs Spur Trail leads right to merge with the Paisley Woods Bicycle Trail and intersect SR 445. Cross the paved road and
enter the recreation area at 0.5 miles for camping, swimming, canoeing,
and parking. Potable water is available.

The FT, however, continues forward to soon cross FR 538. Leave the
rich and varied unburned woods of the recreation area to enter rolling
longleaf-pine and turkey-oak woods with evidence of recent fires. At
mile 10.1, cross paved Lake CR 445. By mile 10.8, the forest has transi-
tioned to mature sand-pine scrub. A younger sand-pine scrub grows on
trail-right, then on both sides of the trail, but this adds up to very few
shade-bearing, mature sand pines overhead. The forest thickens, though,
before emerging onto SR 19 at mile 12.3. Across the road is trailside
parking. The FT crosses SR 19 and enters a mature forest, but there is a

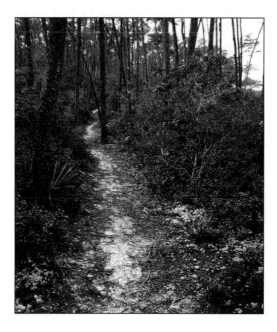

Ocala National Forest,
sand pine scrub

sun-whipped area just to the left. A proliferation of holly dominates the forest understory. This shrubby tree grows bright red berries, seen in the cooler months.

Pass a small sink on trail-left at 12.7 miles. Cross CR 9277, Railroad Grade Road, at 13.0 miles. Soon reach the first wet prairie ringed in live oak, Summit Pond. Live oak and longleaf pines often are found in the moister, more fertile soils. Keep north as the woods briefly revert back to sand-pine scrub before reaching an attractive sizable pond at mile 13.9. There are potential campsites around this quiet locale.

Swing around the north end of the pond to enter sand pine hills again. The trees here have reached their maturity and are beginning to fall. Sand pines are a short-lived species—after 50–70 years or so, the trees begin to succumb to old age and disease. At mile 14.4, intersect the blue-blazed Buck Lake Loop Trail. This trail leads around the east side of Buck Lake past a primitive forest-service campground. The FT leads around the west side of Buck Lake. Stay left with the orange blazes. At first, the trail is far from Buck Lake, although you can glimpse the water. At mile 15.3, intersect the north end of the Buck Lake Loop Trail. The loop trail leads right 0.1 miles to a pump well for water access.

Stay forward on the FT, soon crossing FR 562-2. Undulate west through a mature sand-pine forest. At mile 15.7, a spur trail leads right to quiet Yearling Pond. Past the pond, the trail skirts some cut-over areas in minimal shade. Swing around another small pond before coming to a blue-blazed spur trail leading to Farles Prairie Campground at mile 16.9. This spur trail leads right a short distance to a working pump well.

Continue forward and shortly cross FR 595-E. The forest reverts to mixed pines before reaching FR 595, at mile 17.2. Cross the sandy road and soon intersect a second blue-blazed spur trail leading to Farles Prairie Campground. Water is a half-mile distant on this spur trail. Beyond the spur trail, numerous ponds and prairies dot the thick forest. Come alongside particularly large prairies on both sides of the trail. Live oaks and longleaf pines thrive along these waters. At mile 18.5, pass through sand-pine woods, to emerge onto even larger watery prairies in half a mile. These prairies, collectively known as Ocala Pond, are very shallow and have pines growing sporadically among them. Vistas stretch far in this Florida prairie land.

At mile 20.1, turn away from the shallow prairies, keeping north and rolling through sand-pine woods. Intersect FR 599 at mile 20.8. Stay in sand pine and roller coaster through some of the Ocala's most exceptional hills. Drop to a small prairie at mile 22.0 and re-enter sand-pine woods. The trail enters one final prairie region at mile 22.8. The moister, lower area transitions to live oaks, maples, and palms, culminating in a boardwalk crossing over a wet area at mile 23.3. Leave the wet area just before reaching paved SR 40 at mile 23.5.

Cross SR 40 and head north into the south end of the Juniper Prairie Wilderness. The orange-blazed path soon turns west to roughly parallel SR 40 through a mixed pine forest with an oak and palmetto understory. Leave the wilderness at 24.1 miles to enter the Juniper Springs Recreation Area, which has a campground with hot showers, pay phone, and camp store with limited supplies. Cross the paved entrance road to the campground at 24.7 miles, ending this section of the FT.

# Ocala National Forest, Juniper Springs to Salt Springs Island

| | |
|---|---|
| **Length:** | 18.4 miles |
| **Trail Condition:** | Good |
| **Highs:** | Juniper Prairie Wilderness, vistas, Hidden Pond, Hopkins Prairie |
| **Lows:** | Sun exposure, loose sand |
| **Season:** | Late fall to spring |
| **Difficulty:** | Moderate |
| **Use:** | Moderate, heavier near Juniper Springs Recreation Area and Hopkins Prairie |
| **Tips:** | Have hat and sunscreen ready for this open section of trail |
| **Campsites:** | 3.7, 5.0, 10.1, and 15.9 miles |

**JUNIPER SPRINGS TRAILHEAD:** From Ocala, drive east on SR 40 for 28 miles to Juniper Springs Recreation Area, on your left. The FT starts on the entrance road to the recreation area. Hikers can choose to park their auto inside the recreation area for a fee.

**SALT SPRINGS ISLAND TRAILHEAD:** From Ocala, drive east on SR 40 for 12 miles to Marion CR 314. Turn left on CR 314 and follow it 15.4 miles to paved FR 88. Turn right on FR 88 and follow it for 0.4 miles to the FT. There is parking on the left side of the road, just before the FT crosses FR 88.

This section of FT passes through the rugged Juniper Prairie Wilderness, land of the sand-pine scrub, ponds, and prairies. The FT receives less maintenance on this section, so the hiker will step over logs and under low-lying oak limbs. Most old jeep roads are grown over, but there will be confusing points—stay with the orange blazes. The trail also passes through low-slung pine scrub, where the sun blazes down from above. Juniper Prairie is also where bears roam along Whiskey Creek. Pats Island reveals its past, and the cool waters of Hidden Pond await your arrival. The tops of hills and prairies allow surprising views. Once past Juniper Prairie, the FT passes through a pleasant woodland to reach Hopkins Prairie, the largest in the Ocala. There is a campground and good vistas along this stretch. The FT then leaves the large wetland for a region of smaller prairies to enter a longleaf pine–wiregrass woodland once prevalent over Florida and the Gulf states. This rolling land of towering longleaf pines and knee-high wiregrass offers vistas of its own. This part of the FT deserves more recognition for its beauty.

Camping areas with water access can be found at 3.7, 5.0, 10.1, and 15.9 miles.

❊    ❊    ❊

Start this segment of the FT by walking down the Juniper Springs Recreation Area access road and turning right onto the FT, starting west in a sand-pine forest. At 0.4 miles, enter a low, burned-over oak scrub with an occasional tall sand pine. This section is exposed, but this exposure allows vistas of this hilly terrain. A young forest like this is essential for the perpetuation of species such as the scrub jay and gopher tortoise, which are rapidly losing habitat.

Turn north and briefly enter a mature sand-pine forest before turning back east. At mile 1.1, enter the Juniper Prairie Wilderness. The trail narrows as it passes through sand-pine scrub in many stages of succession. Hike through an open pine-flatwood environment at mile 2.1, to view the first of many prairies and ponds.

Pass some conspicuous palms at mile 2.6 and step over a prairie outflow on a homemade log bridge. Emerge onto a low sand-pine scrub before descending to Whiskey Creek. Cross this perennial stream on a plank footbridge at mile 3.7. The woods are thicker here, with several campsites in the area as well as frequent signs of bears.

The FT keeps north and emerges onto a low pine scrub with many dead snags rising from its flanks. Top out on a hill with good views in all directions. The trail then swings around a small sink before reaching Hidden Pond, a good swimming hole, at mile 5.0. A campsite in the oaks lies on the far side of the pond. The FT, however, stays to the right of the pond and re-enters young scrub. Climb away from Hidden Pond and keep north to gain some shade from a patchwork forest at mile 5.2. The FT briefly merges with, then crosses an old jeep road. Keep the large prairie to your left. The trail turns away from the large prairie at mile 5.6, and primarily stays in an oak forest as it zigzags between scattered ponds and small prairies.

Leave the primary prairie area at mile 6.4 and undulate through a mature sand-pine wood. Reach one more small prairie area at mile 7.0. Climb up a hill to a signed trail junction at mile 7.4. Here, a spur trail leads right for 0.6 miles to Pats Island and the Long Cemetery. Historic Pats Island was romanticized in Marjorie Kinnan Rawlings's novel *The Yearling*. This book captured life in this area during the pioneer days according to Pats Island resident Calvin Long, whom Rawlings interviewed. *The Yearling* was later made into a famous movie starring Gregory Peck that was actually filmed on Pats Island. From the cemetery, the spur trail turns left and heads 0.3 miles to a large, dry sinkhole.

Back at the FT, continue forward from the signed junction, entering a longleaf-pine wood. Pass the Yearling Trail, which has come from SR 19, before leaving the Juniper Prairie Wilderness and reaching FR 10 at mile 8.1. Cross the forest road and enter an oak and sand pine forest. The trail meanders north to pass a sink just before emerging onto FR 86 at mile 9.0.

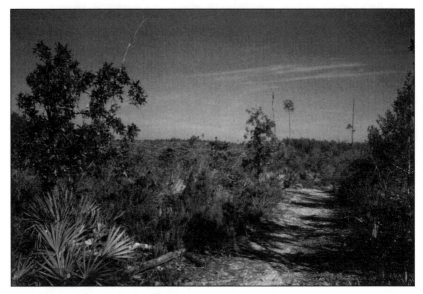

Ocala National Forest, Juniper Prairie

Cross FR 86 and enter the edge of the Hopkins Prairie Recreation Area. Pass to the right of a chilly swimming hole through oak woodland draped in Spanish moss. There will be views of Hopkins Prairie. At mile 9.6, cross the Hopkins Prairie campground access road, FR 86-F. Stay with the orange blazes as the path winds among jeep trails behind the campground. Emerge onto Hopkins Prairie at mile 10.1. The FT turns abruptly to the right. To your left is Hopkins Prairie campground, which has pump well water, toilets, campsites, and hiker parking.

Beyond the campground, the FT heads north along the edge of Hopkins Prairie on an old jeep road. The first of numerous prairie vistas lies through the pines that border the pond-pocked wetland. Another, much smaller broken prairie comes into view on trail-right. The path sometimes winds through the Hopkins Prairie border amid shady oak hammocks as it heads northwest. In other areas, only sky is overhead and hikers will be exposed to the elements above and loose sand below. At mile 11.9, pass a water monitoring station in the prairie. Shortly thereafter, enter a large stand of tall pines. More views reveal fewer ponds on the north end of the prairie.

At mile 12.8, the trail makes a nearly 180° turn back to the southeast around an oak hammock. Continue to swing around the north end of Hopkins Prairie to intersect FR 90-A at mile 13.7. Briefly follow the forest road until it turns right, away from the wetland. Stay left, still paralleling the prairie perimeter.

At mile 14.2, make a sharp right turn into a low oak thicket, leaving Hopkins Prairie and heading northwest. Reach FR 65 at mile 14.5. Cross the sandy road and enter a sand pine scrub forest with a thick understory. Next, cross FR 90 at mile 14.8 and make a noticeable descent. Stay in a rolling sand-pine scrub woodland.

At mile 15.3, the trail winds through numerous small prairies on a pine-oak strand of high ground. Reach a trail junction at mile 15.9. The Salt Springs Spur Trail leads north 2.7 miles to the marina road at the Salt Springs Recreation Area. Salt Springs Recreation Area has a campground with hot showers and a pay phone. The hamlet of Salt Springs is near the recreation area. Supplies are available for long-distance hikers at a small but well stocked grocery store. A pond, located 0.3 miles down this trail, offers water and potential camping.

Keep northwesterly on the FT through a young scrub woodland. Turkey oaks become more abundant. Cross FR 51, and soon come to FR 50 at mile 16.9. On the far side of this road begins the longleaf pine–wiregrass ecosystem. This pine and grass landscape once graced over three million acres in the Southeast. Fire is a necessary and critical component of the longleaf pine–wiregrass forest. Fire suppression, along with development, have played roles in its demise.

This forest has attractive vistas, especially where the terrain begins to undulate. Scattered oak hammocks increase as the path nears FR 88. This is the east edge of Salt Springs Island. Come to paved FR 88 at mile 18.4. From here, it is 17.6 miles to Rodman Dam and the end of the FT in the Ocala National Forest.

# Ocala National Forest, Salt Springs Island to Rodman Dam

| | |
|---|---|
| **Length:** | 17.6 miles |
| **Trail Condition:** | Fair to good |
| **Highs:** | Salt Springs Island, Kerr Island, Penner Ponds, Lake Ocklawaha |
| **Lows:** | Occasional indistinguishable trailbed |
| **Season:** | Late fall to spring |
| **Difficulty:** | Moderate |
| **Use:** | Moderate to low |
| **Tips:** | Consider obtaining water at campgrounds then carrying it to backcountry campsites |
| **Campsites:** | 6.6, 10.0, and 15.4 miles |

**SALT SPRINGS ISLAND TRAILHEAD:** From Ocala, drive east on SR 40 for 12 miles to Marion CR 314. Turn left on CR 314 and follow it 15.4 miles to paved FR 88. Turn right on FR 88 and follow it for 0.4 miles to the FT. There is parking on the left side of the road, just before the FT crosses FR 88.

**RODMAN DAM TRAILHEAD:** From Ocala, drive west on SR 40 for 12 miles to Marion CR 314. Turn left on CR 314 and follow it 18 miles to SR 19. Turn left on SR 19 and follow it north for 11.7 miles to CR 310 (Kirkpatrick Road) and Lake Ocklawaha Recreation Area. Turn left on CR 310 and follow it 3.2 miles to the dam. The parking area is the north side below the dam.

This section of the FT passes over three "islands" in the Ocala: Kerr Island, Salt Springs Island, and Riverside Island. These islands are not surrounded by water in the traditional sense, but are islands of fertile soil, supporting rich stands of longleaf and slash pine, surrounded by the more sterile soils, which support the sand-pine scrub environment so prevalent in the Ocala.

This final, most northern segment of the FT in the Ocala National Forest rolls over Riverside Island, with its attractive pine stands, then passes Penner Ponds, the last prairie/pond complex in the forest. Finally, the FT reaches Lake Ocklawaha, an impoundment that is part of the now defunct Cross Florida Barge Canal project. Nonetheless, the lakeside scenery is attractive and the land remote before the path leaves the national forest, ending up on the far side of Rodman Dam. This section of the FT is used less than in other Ocala locations, and thus offers more opportunities for solitude, even though the path does cross some roads. Backcountry campsites with water are limited to areas near small ponds. Consider camping at Grassy Pond or Lake Delancy campgrounds, or get water from the campgrounds and camp along the trail. The islands of this trail have attractive potential camping areas but no water.

Camping areas with water can be found at 6.6, 10.0, and 15.4 miles.

❈   ❈   ❈

Start this segment of the FT by leaving FR 88 and heading northwest. Enter the eastern end of Salt Springs Island and a longleaf-pine forest with a mixed understory of grass and very young oak scrub. Cross paved CR 314 at 0.4 miles. Continue in a longleaf-pine and turkey-oak forest, with scattered small oak hammocks. Cross FR 19 at mile 1.4.

The trailbed becomes less evident beyond FR 19. Watch for the orange blazes painted on trees while keeping northwest. Cross sandy and small FR 50 at mile 1.7. This road is the northwest border of Salt Springs Island. The forest then reverts to a sand pine scrub. Enter mature sand-pine scrub at 1.9 miles. This especially attractive neck of the woods has a thick understory.

The trail then enters a section of the forest that alternates between older sand pines and younger low scrub. After an extended section of low scrub, reach a high pine woods and FR 63 at mile 3.3. This is the south end of Kerr Island. Keep north into a forest of longleaf pine and turkey oak with a grass and shrub understory. The trailbed here is less evident—stay with the orange blazes.

Cross FR 63 again at mile 3.9. The forest transitions back to sand-pine scrub on the far side of 63. Re-enter Kerr Island at mile 4.3, after crossing FR 63 a third time. At mile 4.8, pass a small land office survey marker from 1928. The FT winds through a stumpy firewood-cutting area before coming to Marion CR 316 at mile 5.2.

Walk into an area of sand pine scrub that is fairly young and doesn't provide much canopy. The sandy trailbed can be loose. Cross FR 88-4 at mile 5.8. The low scrub remains on the far side of FR 88. The rolling nature of the landscape is evident over the woods. Swing past Prairie Pond on your left at mile 6.3, before passing rough FR 88-C. Intersect the short, blue-blazed spur trail to Grassy Pond Campground at mile 6.6. This open and primitive campground is less than desirable. If you must, get water here, then camp on down the line. Be apprised the water supply here has been periodically shut down in the past.

The FT makes a sharp right at a T junction just past the campground. The left-leading trail heads directly to the Grassy Pond pump well. Continue north in low pine scrub, heavy on sand live oak. The canopy resumes at mile 7.2. Deer moss covers the forest floor. Small oak hammocks are scattered over the rolling hills. Pass a private inholding on trail-left, then swing into an attractive longleaf-pine–wiregrass woodland. The forest becomes mixed, with both longleaf-pine and sand-pine scrub forest species represented. Here a real sense of remoteness falls over the land.

Oak increases as the FT nears Lake Delancy. There are some really tall pines in the woods here, too. At mile 9.8, drop down and pass by a dry sink. Soon, cross FR 56. At mile 10.0, a blue-blazed spur trail leads right to Lake Delancy and the south end of primitive Delancy West Campground. Keep forward, crossing FR 85-A. The campground lies off to your right. Intersect FR 75-2 at mile 10.5. The entrance to Delancy West Campground is just to your right. There is a water spigot near the campground host and a pump well is nearby at primitive Delancy East Campground.

The FT leads north from Delancy West Campground into a longleaf-pine forest. Wiregrass, turkey oaks, and dense stands of young live oaks cover the landscape. The dense stands of oaks are sometimes referred to as oak domes; the continuous leaf canopy is lower on the edges and higher in the center. At mile 11.8, the trail cuts through the heart of a shady oak dome.

Beyond this oak dome, longleaf pines begin to dominate the forest. Ferns, flowers, grass, and the occasional saw palmetto rise from the open woodland floor. At mile 12.3, descend alongside a sink. The sink has an open grassy bottom surrounded by large live oaks. It exhibits a lusher look than the surrounding pine forest.

At mile 12.5, cross FR 88-4. Re-enter the pine forest of Riverside Island. Notice all the young longleaf pines. Each has a spindly "trunk" coming up from the ground and is topped with single bulb-like expanse of needles emerging from the top of the plant. These pines are using all their energy to grow their trunk high enough to be able to withstand ground fire caused by lightning. Once they are tall enough, the longleaf pines begin to branch out and gain height.

The longleaf pine–wiregrass forest loses domination as the FT heads north. Turkey oaks and scrub oaks become more prevalent. Cross FR 31 at mile 14.2. Keep rolling over the land and drop down to a sink on your right. Sand pines and longleaf blend past the sink. Cross FR 31-A at mile 15.0, then come to another sandy road with a power line. Leave the pines behind and walk in an oak woodland of varying ages before coming out on FR 77-1 at mile 15.4. Cross FR 77-1. Just across the road, a blue-blazed spur trail leads left to and around Penner Ponds. This is the most northern and final pond/prairie complex in the Ocala that the FT bypasses. Beyond this side trail, which was the old route of the FT, the path has been rerouted and the trailbed is sometimes not evident. Campsites are located along this side trail.

Wind through a mixed forest with intense thickets of sand pine before crossing rough FR 77-A. Pass a tiny pond on your left. Enter a recently cut-over area and come to the north end of the side trail to Penner Ponds at mile 16.2. This far end of Penner Ponds is more desirable, as it is farther from FR 77-1. Turn sharply right and enter a mature sand-pine woods. This area slowly transitions to a live-oak forest draped in Spanish moss before reaching the shores of Lake Ocklawaha. Turn right again, cruising easterly along the shores of the impoundment. Stay alongside the beach-lined shore of Lake Ocklawaha. Emerge onto an open area at mile 16.9, passing a trailside kiosk. Rodman Dam lies to your left. Turn left and walk the dam road to the far side of the dam. At mile 17.6, reach steps that lead to a parking area just below the dam by a dock and the end of the FT in the Ocala National Forest.

## Florida Trail, Ocala National Forest Trail Log

### CLEARWATER LAKE TO JUNIPER SPRINGS

| | | |
|---|---|---|
| 0.0 | 60.7 | Leave Clearwater Lake parking area on access trail |
| 0.2 | 60.5 | Intersect FT, turn left |
| 1.8 | 58.9 | Cross Paisley Road |
| 3.6 | 57.1 | Pass large prairie encircling Duck Pond |
| 4.1 | 56.6 | Leave north end of prairie and enter nearly pure stand of turkey oaks |
| 4.6 | 56.1 | FT passes under major power line |
| 5.2 | 55.5 | Cross Glenn Branch on footbridge, campsites in area |
| 5.7 | 55.0 | Bisect junglesque swamp on long boardwalk |
| 6.2 | 54.5 | Cross FR 539 |
| 6.5 | 54.2 | Pass through small prairie, forest transitions to sand pine |
| 7.8 | 52.9 | Cross FR 538E |
| 8.9 | 51.8 | Long boardwalk over sporadic wet area |
| 9.3 | 51.4 | Intersect Alexander Springs Spur Trail, leads to recreation area with camping, hot showers, pay phone, swimming, and canoeing, FT keeps forward and crosses FR 538 |
| 10.1 | 50.6 | Cross paved Lake CR 445 |
| 10.8 | 49.9 | Forest transitions to mature sand-pine scrub |
| 12.3 | 48.4 | Cross paved SR 19, trailside parking |
| 12.7 | 48.0 | Pass small sink on trail-left |
| 13.0 | 47.7 | Cross Railroad Grade Road |
| 13.9 | 46.8 | Attractive sizable pond, potential campsites |
| 14.4 | 46.3 | Intersect blue-blazed Buck Lake Loop Trail, FT stays left around Buck Lake |
| 15.3 | 45.4 | Intersect north end of Buck Lake Loop Trail, pump well 0.1 miles to right on loop trail, FT keeps forward, soon crossing FR 562-2 |
| 15.7 | 45.0 | Side trail lead to Yearling Pond |
| 16.9 | 43.8 | Spur trail leads to Farles Prairie Campground, pump well water, and primitive camping, FT keeps forward to cross FR 595-E |
| 17.2 | 43.5 | Cross sandy FR 595, soon reach second blue-blazed spur trail leading right to Farles Prairie Campground |
| 18.5 | 42.2 | Sand pine woods between large prairies collectively known as Ocala Pond |
| 20.1 | 40.6 | Turn away from prairies |
| 20.8 | 39.9 | Cross FR 599, roller coaster through sand-pine hills |
| 22.0 | 38.7 | Drop to small prairie |

## Florida Trail, Ocala National Forest Trail Log *(continued)*

| | | |
|---|---|---|
| **23.3** | **37.4** | Boardwalk over wet area |
| **23.5** | **37.2** | Cross paved SR 40, enter south end of Juniper Prairie Wilderness |
| **24.1** | **36.6** | Enter Juniper Springs Recreation Area, campground with hot showers, pay phone, and camp store with limited supplies |
| **24.7** | **36.0** | Cross paved recreation area entrance road |

### JUNIPER SPRINGS TO SALT SPRINGS ISLAND

| | | |
|---|---|---|
| **25.1** | **35.6** | Enter low burned over oak scrub |
| **25.8** | **34.9** | Re-enter Juniper Prairie Wilderness |
| **26.8** | **33.9** | Open pine flatwoods |
| **27.3** | **33.4** | Pass conspicuous palms and step over prairie outflow on boardwalk |
| **28.4** | **32.3** | Cross Whiskey Creek on plank footbridge, campsites in area |
| **29.7** | **31.0** | Hidden Pond, good swimming hole, campsite on far side of pond |
| **30.3** | **30.4** | FT turns away from large prairie, pass through scattered ponds and prairies |
| **32.1** | **28.6** | Spur trail leads right to Pats Island and Long Cemetery |
| **32.8** | **27.9** | Cross FR 10 |
| **33.7** | **27.0** | Cross FR 86, pass by deep swimming hole on edge of Hopkins Prairie Recreation Area |
| **34.3** | **26.4** | Cross Hopkins Prairie campground access road, FR 86-F |
| **34.8** | **25.9** | Emerge onto Hopkins Prairie, primitive Hopkins Prairie Campground to left, pump well water, FT turns right along edge of prairie |
| **36.6** | **24.1** | Pass water monitoring station on edge of Hopkins Prairie |
| **37.5** | **23.2** | Make acute turn to southeast in oak hammock |
| **38.4** | **22.3** | Intersect FR 90-A, briefly follow road |
| **38.9** | **21.8** | Make sharp right turn in oak thicket, leave Hopkins Prairie |
| **39.2** | **21.5** | Cross sandy FR 65 |
| **39.5** | **21.2** | Cross FR 90, make noticeable descent |
| **40.0** | **20.7** | FT winds through pine-oak strand of high ground |
| **40.6** | **20.1** | Intersect Salt Springs Spur Trail, it leads 2.7 miles to Salt Springs Recreation Area, campground, hot showers, and pay phone, nearby hamlet of Salt Springs has small but well-stocked grocery store |
| **41.6** | **19.1** | Cross FR 50 after crossing FR 51, enter longleaf pine–wiregrass ecosystem broken with oak hammocks |
| **43.1** | **17.6** | Reach paved FR 88, enter Salt Springs Island |

## Florida Trail, Ocala National Forest Trail Log *(continued)*

### SALT SPRINGS ISLAND TO RODMAN DAM

| | | |
|---|---|---|
| **43.5** | **17.2** | Cross paved CR 314, continue in longleaf-pine and turkey-oak woods |
| **44.5** | **16.2** | Cross FR 19, trailbed becomes more faint |
| **44.8** | **15.9** | Cross FR 50, leave Salt Springs Island, forest reverts to sand-pine scrub |
| **46.4** | **14.3** | Enter Kerr Island after crossing FR 63, area of longleaf pine |
| **47.0** | **13.7** | Cross FR 63 again, area of sand pine scrub |
| **47.4** | **13.3** | Re-enter Kerr Island after crossing FR 63 yet again |
| **47.9** | **12.8** | Pass land office survey marker from 1928, enter firewood-cutting area |
| **48.3** | **12.4** | Cross Marion CR 316, leave Kerr Island for good |
| **48.9** | **11.8** | Cross FR 88-4, rolling landscape covered in sand pine scrub |
| **49.4** | **11.3** | Swing past Prairie Pond, cross rough FR 88-C |
| **49.7** | **10.8** | Intersect blue-blazed spur trail leading to primitive Grassy Pond Campground, unreliable pump well at campground, make sharp right at T junction |
| **50.3** | **10.2** | Forest becomes canopied again |
| **52.9** | **7.8** | Pass by dry sink and soon cross FR 56 |
| **53.1** | **7.6** | Spur trail leads right to primitive Delancy West Campground, soon cross FR 85-A |
| **53.6** | **7.1** | Cross FR 75-2, Delancy West Campground to right, water spigot near campground host, pump well at nearby Delancy East Campground |
| **54.9** | **5.8** | Trail cuts through shady oak dome amid longleaf-pine forest |
| **55.4** | **5.3** | Descend alongside a sink |
| **55.6** | **5.1** | Enter Riverside Island after crossing FR 88-4, area of young longleaf pines |
| **57.3** | **3.4** | Cross FR 31, rolling landscape |
| **58.1** | **2.6** | Cross FR 31-A |
| **58.5** | **2.2** | Cross FR 77-1, blue-blazed spur trail leads left around Penner Ponds, campsite along spur trail, FT keeps forward and crosses rough FR 77-A |
| **59.3** | **1.4** | Intersect north end of spur trail circling Penner Ponds, FT turns sharply right |
| **60.0** | **0.7** | Enter open area after reaching shores of Lake Ocklawaha, turn left on dam road |

## Florida Trail, Ocala National Forest Trail Log *(continued)*

**60.7    0.0**    Reach steps leading to parking area below Rodman Dam, end of FT in Ocala National Forest

## Ocala National Forest Trail Information

Ocala National Forest
www.r8web/florida/forests/ocala.htm

Seminole Ranger District
40929 State Road 19
Umatilla, Florida 32784
(352) 669-3153

Lake George Ranger District
17147 East Highway 40
Silver Springs, Florida 34488
(352) 625-2520

# Florida Trail,
# Apalachicola National Forest

The Apalachicola is Florida's largest national forest. It encompasses a wide swath of the panhandle, from Tallahassee in the east to the Apalachicola River in the west. Within these confines, visitors will find sand hills, sinkholes, lakes, pinelands, blackwater streams, spring-fed ponds, rich swamps, and rivers. The vast amounts of water that flow through this land feed the rich estuaries of the Gulf. The flora along these waterways—cypress, black gum, titi, sweetbay magnolia, and more—act as a filter to cleanse the water that produces vast amounts of shellfish off the Florida coast. Tall longleaf woods mixed with oaks and occasional hardwood hammocks provide food and cover for deer and scrub jays alike.

Hikers will enjoy this 65-mile section of the FT that bisects the national forest. The path passes through nearly every environment the Apalachicola has to offer—longleaf-pine flatwoods, hills cloaked in oaks, the beautiful watershed of the Sopchoppy River, and the deep swamps of Bradwell Bay—most of it in solitude. A sense of solitude continues in the western half of the forest where creeks abound, such as Coxes Branch. Visit the deserted community of Vilas, then enter a place of hills, lakes, and savannas before leaving the forest.

There are several unique areas the FT passes through, including savannas—grassy plains that are both flood and fire tolerant—and the Bradwell Bay Wilderness, with nearly 25,000 acres of open pinelands and some of the deepest swamps in the entire forest. Hikers may also get a chance to see some of the forests more unusual residents, including the carnivorous pitcher plant, which captures insects and absorbs them as food.

Hikers should always keep in mind that resupply points are nonexistent, but making the 65-mile trek is possible without resupply. Backcountry campsites are numerous along the rivers and streams of the forest. There are also a few designated backcountry campsites developed by the Florida Trail Association. The FT also passes two primitive forest-service campgrounds.

# Apalachicola National Forest, Medart to Bradwell Bay

| | |
|---|---|
| **Length:** | 12.7 miles |
| **Trail Condition:** | Good |
| **Highs:** | Sopchoppy River, old growth magnolias, solitude |
| **Lows:** | Steep sandy ravines |
| **Season:** | Fall through spring |
| **Difficulty:** | Moderate |
| **Use:** | Low, moderate along Sopchoppy River |
| **Tips:** | Take your time along the Sopchoppy River |
| **Campsites:** | Numerous |

**MEDART TRAILHEAD:** From the Wakulla County courthouse in Crawfordville, drive 8.2 miles south on US 319 to the FT Medart trailhead, on your right. There is a parking area here.

**BRADWELL BAY TRAILHEAD:** From the Wakulla Ranger Station on US 319 south of Tallahassee, head south on US 319 for 3.8 miles to Crawfordville and the Wakulla County Courthouse. Turn right at the stoplight just before the courthouse, on Arran Road (Wakulla CR 368). Arran Road turns into Forest Highway 13. Follow Arran Road for 4.6 miles to FR 365. Turn left on FR 365 and follow it for 2.9 miles to FR 348. Turn right on FR 348 and follow it for 2.5 miles to FR 329. Turn left on FR 329 and follow it for 0.4 miles to the Bradwell Bay Wilderness trailhead, on your right.

Hikers on the Apalachicola National Forest portion of the FT head northwest from US 319 to traverse a seldom-visited land, following mostly footpaths over rolling pine woods to reach a lush woodland with old-growth magnolias and other trees. The trail drops down to the Sopchoppy River valley and provides some of the best of the FT. Here the path meanders beneath live oaks alongside the blackwater stream, where huge cypress trees with oddly-shaped "knees" line the waterway. Side streams cut deep gullies, making for a lot of ups and downs. The FT emerges onto a forest road to end this section near Bradwell Bay Wilderness.

Camping areas can be found near most streams the trail crosses.

❊    ❊    ❊

Start this segment of the FT by leaving US 319 behind, passing a trail register and immediately entering an eye-pleasing forest of pine, live oak, and laurel oak. At 0.3 miles, come to a long and winding boardwalk over a low area of bay, titi, and cypress. Continue on a footpath in a more open forest. Come alongside FR 356, then cross it at mile 1.0. Drop down off a hill and near a thicket before turning back toward the forest road.

At mile 1.4, reach a longleaf-pine plantation, then drop down to a titi thicket. The next thicket, with a wide stream beneath the dark canopy, is crossed at mile 1.9 on a plank bridge. Turn right and walk the margin dividing the stream just crossed and pine woods. The land here is low sand hills of pine and turkey oak broken by titi thickets. Occasionally, the trail will take forest roads for short sections. The faint footbed testifies to the infrequent use of the trail.

Step over a blackwater stream at mile 3.9. Turn left immediately past the stream, entering a young, dense longleaf-pine plantation, and cross a jeep track among taller pines. At mile 4.7, come to a turkey oak stand atop a hill. Drop down to cross FR 321 at mile 5.3. The next section makes a lot of twists and turns—pay close attention here. First, cross FR 321-C at mile 5.5, staying in thick woods, then pass under a power line. Return to FR 321-C and span a stream on a forest road bridge. Immediately past the bridge, enter the forest to the right and settle down to woods hiking. Pass through a pine plantation before reaching a mature pineland at mile 6.6. This area is favored by red-cockaded woodpeckers, as is evidenced by numerous pines circled with white paint stripes, indicating woodpecker holes bored into trees that serve as nests.

At mile 7.2, reach an area with many live oaks and laurel oaks with a brushy understory. This leads into a low area with many big trees. Of special note are the old growth sweetbay magnolia trees. Commonly known as bay trees or swamp magnolia, these trees keep their leaves year-round, extending from South Florida northward to Massachusetts and westward to Texas. Look around for other large trees, such as red maple and tulip poplars. Stay in lush woods, mostly deciduous trees, before entering one last section of big magnolias, then intersect FR 365 at mile 8.1. The FT crosses the road and continues northwest through shady woods.

Drop down to the banks of the Sopchoppy River and head upstream a short distance, reaching FR 346 at mile 8.6. Turn left on the sandy vehicle road and immediately span the Sopchoppy on a wooden bridge. Follow the forest road for 0.2 miles. The FT then re-enters the woods on the right, along the west bank of the Sopchoppy River. This section of the FT was once known as the Apalachicola Trail.

Immediately cross under a power line, then cross a small creek on a plank bridge at mile 9.1. Keep north through rich woods of water oak, sweetgum, red maple, and pine. Cross a feeder stream on a footbridge and swing around an inholding, coming to the banks of the Sopchoppy River at 9.4 miles. At this point, the FT is 30 feet above the river, though over the next couple miles bluff heights range between 20 and 50 feet above the river. Observe the huge cypress trees with their strange "knees" along the river. Soon come to a roller coaster–like section of trail, dropping down into and emerging out of the gullies of numerous feeder streams as you continue along the river's bluffline. Most of the gullies flow only during rainy periods.

At times, the FT turns away from the bluffline instead of following the sharp bends of the Sopchoppy. The footbed is generally narrow. Sand live oak, palmetto, live oak, and holly border the river and trail. Continue to undulate, crossing cypress and bamboo filled ravines.

Leave the riverside at mile 10.1, passing through a titi-bay forest, and climbing onto pine flatwoods. Soon, pick up a jeep track on high ground. Turkey oaks grow here. Veer right, away from the jeep track at mile 10.8, and drop steeply down to Monkey Creek. Span this large stream on a footbridge. Rise to a pine plantation and walk among the rows of evergreens. Reach the riverbank at mile 11.2, once more enjoying the superlative beauty of the Sopchoppy River. Continue to climb up and down the steep ravines, stepping over a perennial feeder stream in 0.2 miles. Swamps occasionally appear—the trail effectively straddles the bluff between the Sopchoppy on the right and the swamps on the left. At times the path drops directly alongside the coffee-colored waters of the river.

Pass another perennial stream at mile 12.4. Soon, the trail circumvents a wide swamp. Cross a series of boardwalk footbridges before climbing to a dry open area, which is the official Sopchoppy River back-country campsite. Past the camping area, pick up a wide trail that leads to FR 329. A bridge over the Sopchoppy lies just to the right. The FT, however, turns left and follows FR 329 for 0.2 miles to the Bradwell Bay Wilderness trailhead, the end of this segment. From here, it is 19.0 miles to Porter Lake on the FT.

## Apalachicola National Forest, Bradwell Bay to Porter Lake

| | |
|---|---|
| **Length:** | 19.0 miles |
| **Trail Condition:** | Fair to good |
| **Highs:** | Federally designated wilderness, blackwater river |
| **Lows:** | Poorly marked mucky path, minimal trailbed, miles of swamp walking |
| **Season:** | Fall through spring |
| **Difficulty:** | Moderate to difficult, swamp sections can be very difficult in high water |
| **Tips:** | Prepare for wet feet, guaranteed |
| **Campsites:** | Numerous except in second half of Bradwell Bay Wilderness |

**BRADWELL BAY TRAILHEAD:** From the Wakulla Ranger Station on US 319 south of Tallahassee, head south on US 319 for 3.8 miles to Crawfordville and the Wakulla County Courthouse. Turn right at the stoplight just before the courthouse, on Arran Road (Wakulla CR 368). Follow Arran Road for 4.6 miles to FR 365(Along the way, Arran Road turns into Forest Highway 13.). Turn left on FR 365 and follow it for 2.9 miles to FR 348. Turn right on FR 348 and follow it for 2.5 miles to FR 329. Turn left on FR 329 and follow it for 0.4 miles to the Bradwell Bay Wilderness trailhead, on your right.

**PORTER LAKE TRAILHEAD:** From junction of SR 263 and SR 20 near Tallahassee, drive west on SR 20 for 17.5 miles to Leon CR 375.

(Leon CR 375 turns into SR 375). Stay on 375 for 17.4 miles to Forest Highway 13. Turn right on FH 13 and follow it for 1.2 miles to Porter Lake Campground on your left. This section of the FT leaves from the campground itself.

This segment of the FT heads across the Bradwell Bay Wilderness and beyond to the banks of the Ocklockonee River. The FT traverses through completely different sections of the wilderness. It begins where the sun beats down over scant pines standing among palmetto prairies. Suddenly, the FT enters miles of wet, shady cypress-and-hardwood swamps with very little dry land. The path then emerges onto an area of dead, standing pines ravaged by wildfire. Beyond the wilderness, the path remains wet, cruising through row-cropped slash pines—rows were dug and the slash pines planted on the higher ground between the rows in pursuit of better growing conditions. Finally, a little road walking is necessary, circumventing the wide floodplain swamp surrounding the Ocklockonee River, to end at Porter Lake Campground.

Camping flats are abundant through the section, with the exception of the second half of the Bradwell Bay Wilderness area.

❁    ❁    ❁

Leave the Bradwell Bay parking area and enter the nearly 25,000-acre Bradwell Bay Wilderness, the largest wilderness in Florida. This wide, wet depression was named for a hunter who was lost for days in the swamps and thickets of the area. After passing through the wilderness in its entirety, you will be appreciative of the orange blazes that mark the FT here. Leave the trailhead and trace an old road, flanked by a canal, through mixed flatwoods of pine, sand live oak, and water oak. Pass a trailside registration kiosk, then bridge a small creek surrounded by bamboo. Emerge into an open, sun-splashed brush plain, reaching pine woods at 0.8 miles. This wilderness is home to black bears—you may see their acorn-laden scat on the path.

Easily span a second creek on the remnants of a road bridge at mile 1.0. The trailside here is a mixed forest of oaks and pines. At mile 1.4, enter a palmetto-gallberry plain over which the blackened trunks of burned pines tower. Ponds border the trail. At mile 2.0, reach a stand of live oaks on trail-left, which serves as a potential camping area, though water is not directly available nearby. Notice the increase in turkey oaks. Just a short distance past the live oaks, leave the roadbed and make an acute turn left onto another, less obvious roadbed. This left turn is signed. The roadbed the trail has been following continues north and becomes an unmaintained trail kept open by hunters and game.

A preponderance of spindly pines crowd the path, giving way to a brush field stark with standing dead trees. The trailbed here is likely to be crowded with undergrowth and wet in places. Wilderness trails are less-maintained by design, to make the experience more challenging and rustic. Expect thick brush and fallen trees throughout Bradwell Bay.

At mile 3.1, enter a titi thicket centered on a six-foot-wide stream that must be crossed without a bridge. Cross a pine island and shortly bisect a titi-bay-cypress thicket. Come out onto a brush plain sparsely wooded in pine. Quickly enter another titi thicket and continue on wet trail bordered in pond pine, more evidence of a high water table. Swing to the south around a saucer-shaped depression at mile 3.9 and enter a huge palmetto prairie. Occasional orange tape is tied to brush, indicating the trail. Also, watch the footbed below for assurances you are on the path. After a half mile, a few trees begin to appear trailside, but the terrain is open more often than not. Pass a small pond at mile 4.6. Briefly traverse another bay thicket with a small stream running through it before reaching a trail junction in an open area at mile 4.9. A blue-blazed spur trail leads left 0.5 miles through palmetto prairie and turkey oaks to reach FR 329 at Monkey Creek.

The FT continues right, turning onto an old jeep road and entering pine flatwoods at 5.0 miles. Keep west in these pine flatwoods and descend into a titi-cypress swamp, crossing a feeder stream of Monkey Creek at 6.0 miles. Emerge onto a palmetto plain with a few scattered pond pines and longleaf pines. The trail is brushy in spots.

Drop down again to ford Monkey Creek at mile 6.4. There once was a bridge here and there may be one in the future, but by now you have given up hope of keeping your boots dry. Stay in a lush shady woodland on the far side of Monkey Creek. This lush forest gives way to tall longleaf-pine woodland. Watch here as the trail unexpectedly turns sharply right and passes through a swamp at mile 7.1. Climb back to pine woods, the last significant dry ground for over a mile and a half, and intersect a blue-blazed spur trail at mile 7.3. The spur trail leads left 150 yards to FR 329.

Descend into a wet area of bay, pond pine, and cypress. This swamp section is broken by one little area of pines 0.7 miles distant. Before the water is finished dribbling off your legs atop this little pine island, enter another swamp that goes unbroken a long while. Look down to check the water flow of the swamp—the water should flow against you. Emerge onto a larger pine island at mile 9.0. This area was burned and has many standing dead trees. Savor the dry ground here and realize this provides the last viable camping area for miles.

Enter a long swamp. Overhead are old growth trees—pine, cypress, and gum. Look for a huge double-trunked cypress on trail-left at mile 9.6. At mile 10.2, the still waters can be mucky in an area of deciduous swamp trees. More open sections of water can and will easily top your knees. Roots, submerged logs, and deep pockets make for uneven and rough going. In times past, ropes have been strung between trees for easier passage. Be very careful and have the most critical items in your pack waterproofed. In times of high water, you will be submerged to your waist. Put to rest any concerns about leeches; your biggest hazard will be keeping your footing.

By mile 10.5, the water has become more shallow, but the footing is still very uneven. There are scattered places to rest or sit down. At mile 11.2, the FT enters an area where the swamp hardwoods are thin. Pass through one more deep section before emerging onto dry land and picking up a logging tram with canals on both sides of it. The dry land is open. Continuing to follow the tram bed, once again enter into a brief section of swamp. Climb out to a pine forest. The majority of the trees are living and the trail is mostly dry, but parts of the area have been burned and some trail sections are still wet. The FT follows the old tram road, which veers right at mile 12.5. At mile 12.7, drop down to one more titi thicket and for one last wet-footed wilderness walk before coming to FR 314 at mile 13.1.

Leave the Bradwell Bay Wilderness at FR 314. Turn right and walk along the built-up forest road for 0.6 miles, passing a beekeeper's hive on your left. Leave the forest road and turn left onto a four-wheel drive track through a pine plantation with canals cut along it. The water table is quite high here and the path can be wet. At mile 14.0, the FT leaves the jeep trail and veers right into pines with an understory of gallberry and some palmetto.

Come to a titi-cypress thicket and plunge into the water. There is just enough high ground around to attempt to keep your feet dry, but sooner or later they are going to get wet. Leave the titi thicket and reach a row-cropped pine plantation. For the hiker it means wet feet even though the trail passes through a pine plantation, which usually means dry walking.

At mile 14.7, the FT reaches a non-numbered but sporadically maintained forest road. Follow this road forward to FR 388 at mile 15.0. Turn right on FR 388 and follow it for 0.6 miles to double orange blazes. Leave the forest road left and enter another wet pine plantation on an ultra-rough four-wheel-drive track. Brush such as yaupon lines the path. Pass through a pine-titi-bay thicket on a side trail, avoiding deep water on the jeep road. At mile 16.1, the trail sidetracks again in a titi-cypress thicket. A blackwater creek flows through the center of this thicket. Stay the course westerly, making detours only around muddy water on the jeep track. Emerge onto SR 375 at mile 16.8. Turn right and follow the paved road north over Smith Creek.

If you are a member of the Florida Trail Association, you can leave SR 375 at mile 17.5, veering left and walking through private land for 0.9 miles until the trail emerges onto FH 13. All others should stay on SR 375 for 0.5 miles to FH 13. Turn left on FH 13, and follow it for 1.2 miles until the FT emerges onto FH 13, just before the bridge over the Ocklockonee River. Span the Ocklockonee on the bridge, passing another bridge over Porter Lake and drop left off the road after 0.6 miles to Porter Lake Campground, ending this segment of the FT at mile 19.0. From here it is 19.1 miles northwest to Vilas on the FT.

# Apalachicola National Forest, Porter Lake to Vilas

| | |
|---|---|
| **Length:** | 19.1 miles |
| **Trail Condition:** | Good |
| **Highs:** | Numerous streams, wiregrass prairies, former turpentining community |
| **Lows:** | Wobbly footbridges |
| **Season:** | Fall through spring |
| **Difficulty:** | Moderate |
| **Use:** | Low to moderate |
| **Tips:** | Consider using designated backcountry campsites spread along this section |
| **Campsites:** | Numerous |

**PORTER LAKE TRAILHEAD:** From junction of SR 263 and SR 20 near Tallahassee, drive west on SR 20 for 17.5 miles to Leon CR 375. (Leon CR 375 turns into SR 375). Stay on 375 for 17.4 miles to FH 13. Turn right on FH 13 and follow it for 1.2 miles to Porter Lake Campground on your left. This section of the FT leaves from the campground itself.

**VILAS TRAILHEAD:** From the Apalachicola Ranger Station in Bristol, head west on SR 20 for 0.4 miles to SR 12. Turn left on SR 12 and follow it for 13 miles to FR 108. Turn left on FR 108 and follow it 3 miles to FR 112. Turn right on FR 112 and follow it 4.5 miles to SR 65. Turn left on SR 65 and follow it 0.4 miles to FR 120. Turn right on FR 120 and follow it 0.2 miles to the trailhead on the left just after the railroad tracks.

This segment of the FT is ideal for backpacking. The combination of campsite availability and varied forest ecosystems adds practicality and interest to the solitude-filled hike. The pathway heads west from Porter Lake, crossing numerous streams, sometimes on footbridges and sometimes on road bridges. A variety of environments lie along the way. Pine palmetto flatwoods give way to titi, cypress, and hardwoods along streams and swamps. Extensive prairies of wiregrass, dotted with longleaf pine, lie in the middle of this section.

Numerous camping sites, including three official FT campsites, Jewell Tower, Sapling Head, and Vilas, are scattered alongside the trail. Expect to have little company.

❁   ❁   ❁

Leave Porter Lake Campground from near the rest rooms, heading west in a thick woodland of water oak, magnolia, and loblolly pine. Pass a trail registration station, crossing a swamp on a footlog at 0.2 miles. Keep along the path and cross FH 13 at 0.7 miles. Turn north in a longleaf-pine woodland, picking up a jeep trail. Cross a small branch at 0.9 miles on a footlog. The path climbs a bit and enters a young pine plantation. Leave the jeep trail. Straddle the perimeter between longleaf pines on your left and a floodplain marsh on your right.

The FT spans another stream on a footlog at mile 1.7, and emerges onto a longleaf-wiregrass-palmetto woodland, paralleling the stream just crossed. At mile 2.0, in an open field, the trail veers off to the right. Soon, cross another stream on a footlog. Climb onto a slash pine plantation. Keep up with the orange blazes, as the FT changes jeep tracks frequently. Not only is this area laced with jeep trails, but also wet titi thickets and small creeks. That is why the FT follows jeep tracks here— they are often the highest places around.

The FT eventually returns to a footpath, as evidenced by the next section that heads through tulip trees, water oaks, and bay trees. At mile 3.0, cross FR 142, spanning Hickory Branch, then veer left into longleaf-pine woodland. Drop steeply to cross Coxes Branch on an unusual suspension bridge at mile 4.3. Notice the large loblolly pine to which one side of the bridge is attached. Loblolly, which is a Creek Indian word for mud puddle, prefer deep, poorly drained floodplains in the Apalachicola, but will also grow in fertile uplands and old fields.

Continue into a titi-bamboo thicket that follows beside Indian Creek. At mile 4.6, reach the Jewell Tower campsite, marked with a FT sign posted to a tree. Water can be obtained from Indian Creek. Cross paved CR 67 at mile 4.7. Turn right on the road, spanning Indian Creek, then turn left into a hilly area that becomes grown over with turkey oaks, then longleaf pines. Pick up a jeep trail at mile 5.2 and keep west, crossing FR 117 at mile 6.2.

Stay in turkey oak, longleaf pine, and wiregrass, dropping to a wet area of pond pine and cypress, before reaching FR 107 at mile 7.0. Make a westward road walk on this forest road—the only dry footing for miles. Cross the headwaters of Indian Creek, coming to the junction with FR 126 at mile 7.9. Continue forward on FR 107. Pine plantations growing over soaked brush lie alongside the road.

At mile 9.3, on a curve, the FT leaves the road to dive left into thick brush and pine. The woods become increasingly wet, with titi thickets along a creek. Stay in brush, crossing a floodplain and stream on a long plank bridge just before coming to FR175 at mile 10.6. Cross the sandy road, then come to a sign indicating Sapling Head campsite. It is on a spur trail leading right on the far side of a narrow floodplain swamp. The FT, however, continues forward alongside the headwaters of Bay

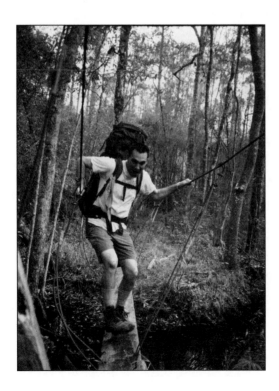

Hiker balancing on
Coxes Branch bridge

Creek. Intersect a jeep trail and make a sharp right, crossing Bay Creek at mile 11.0.

Keep with the jeep trail, passing through a titi thicket and emerging onto an impressive prairie of wiregrass, dotted with longleaf pines. There are good views into the forest beyond. The FT turns sharply right, now as a foot trail, and borders the perimeter of the prairie. A titi thicket lies to your right. Pond pines grow where the wiregrass and titi come together. Leave the longleaf prairie at mile 12.5, dropping into a floodplain swamp, crossing a blackwater stream, and beginning a pattern of alternating between wiregrass prairies and floodplain swamps. This area oozes solitude, even with the crossing of FR 107-B at mile 14.5.

Keep with the swamp-wiregrass-swamp pattern, and bisect Saplin Head Swamp at mile 16.2. Turn north in wiregrass topped with longleaf pines and turkey oaks, coming to FR 107 at mile 17.0. Turn left on FR 107 and span Black Creek on a road bridge. Look for Atlantic white cedar along the fringes of the watercourse. Cross a tributary stream of Black Creek at mile 17.7, then head north on a foot trail, paralleling a feeder stream. Turn away from the feeder stream to dip down through a few titi-bay thickets between pinelands.

At mile 18.9, reach the Vilas campsite, on your right beneath tall pines. Water is available at the last stream crossed. The former community of Vilas lies just beyond the campsite. Vilas' economy and existence was based on the production of turpentine, a sticky substance critical to the shipping industry. Florida had been exporting naval supplies since the early 1740s, when the first schooner left Pensacola for Havana with turpentine, pine pitch, and pine logs. Turpentine was made from the sap of Florida's abundant pines. The sap was collected in clay pots, then boiled and rendered into turpentine, and used to preserve wood and waterproof ships. The town reached it's peak during the 1920s. Look around for relics of that era, but leave them for others to enjoy.

Come to FR 120 and end this segment of the FT at mile 19.1. From here, it is 9.9 miles to Camel Lake campground, and 15.8 miles to SR 12 and the end of the FT through the Apalachicola National Forest at Estiffanulga.

# Apalachicola National Forest, Vilas to Estiffanulga

| | |
|---|---|
| **Length:** | 15.8 miles |
| **Trail Condition:** | Good |
| **Highs:** | Memery Island, numerous creeks, lakes, savannas |
| **Lows:** | Sun exposure, swamps |
| **Season:** | Fall through spring |
| **Difficulty:** | Moderate |
| **Use:** | Low, moderate around Camel Lake campground |
| **Tips:** | Beware of slick wooden footbridges |
| **Campsites:** | Numerous |

**VILAS TRAILHEAD:** From the Apalachicola Ranger Station in Bristol, head west on SR 20 for 0.4 miles to SR 12. Turn left on SR 12 and follow it for 13 miles to FR 108. Turn left on FR 108 and follow it 3 miles to FR 112. Turn right on FR 112 and follow it 4.5 miles to SR 65. Turn left on SR 65 and follow it 0.4 miles to FR 120. Turn right on FR 120 and follow it 0.2 miles to the trailhead on the left just after the railroad tracks.

**ESTIFFANULGA TRAILHEAD:** From the Apalachicola Ranger Station in Bristol, head west on SR 20 for 0.4 miles to SR 12. Turn left on SR 12 and follow it for 10 miles to the FT, which exits the forest on the left side of the road.

This section of the FT traverses numerous environments and offers vertical variation. Leave Vilas and pass along the floodplain of the New River. Beyond here, the trailbed can be wet, as it passes through a full-blown swamp. Climb to higher, drier ground and come to pretty Bonnet Pond, ringed in cypress, and the Trail of Lakes. Head through turkey oaks, then cross perennial stream Big Gully Creek and the cool swamp woods around it. Pass over dry hills and down into a juniper swamp, on to the crystal-clear Camel Lake, a National Forest recreation area and campground. Past

Camel Lake, climb Memery Island, a sandy knob topped in live oaks. Finally, enjoy unique savannas—grassy wetlands where carnivorous pitcher plants thrive among widely scattered pines.

Numerous potential camping spots make this section appealing to backpackers.

❁   ❁   ❁

The FT leaves Vilas, heading west a short distance on FR 120 before crossing over the Apalachicola Northern railroad tracks. The trail then turns left into a tall wood with a marshy footbed. At 0.3 miles, come to SR 65 and turn left, crossing the New River on a road bridge. At 0.7 miles, come to FR 112 and turn right, tracing the sandy road just a short distance before heading right again, away from the road and through a cattle fence paralleling the floodplain swamp of the New River in young longleaf growth. At mile 1.8, drop down along the New River on a wet trail shadowed by tall cypress. When leaving the swamp, look for carnivorous pitcher plants in the trailside grass before climbing to a pine plantation with a brushy understory.

At mile 3.1, come to FR 112-H. Turn right here and cross Hostage Branch on a road bridge. Veer left onto a foot trail that passes through brushy woods with a wet footbed in many spots. At mile 4.2, drop into a full-blown swamp, which extends for a full half mile. Toward the end of this swamp, cut logs provide dry footing, but they are slick, moss-covered, and will make slippage more likely.

At mile 5.5, enter private land—the property boundary is marked. Pass through the private land for 0.3 miles and return to national-forest land, now on little-used FR 108-D. Turkey oaks increase in number. Pass a large field on your right just before crossing FR 108 at mile 6.2. Ahead the forest road splits—take the right fork and follow FR 108-E.

At mile 6.6, reach a trail junction. The south terminus of the Trail of Lakes comes in from the right. Dead ahead is Bonnet Pond. The waterside shores make a good camping locale. Stay left on the FT to follow the shore of Bonnet Pond. Check out the wide-buttressed cypress trees that encircle this small body of water. Pass by another smaller pond before turning away from the water, alongside a wet strand to your left. Circle a normally dry lake bed at mile 7.7, then pick up a straight dug path, that was a firebreak at one time. Drop off the hill and come to FR 105 at mile 8.1. Turn left along the forest road to bridge Big Gully Creek. Leave the road after the creek and turn left again, climbing a hilltop.

Cruise along the hilltop through turkey oak and sand live oak, all the while heading toward Camel Lake. Drop into a thicket at mile 9.0, crossing an unnamed stream on a plank bridge. Continue walking the plank until the trail emerges onto a well-drained pine-oak woodland, soon reaching another plank bridge through a juniper-filled swamp strand. At mile 9.9, come to the side trail leading left to Camel Lake Recreation Area, with camping, fishing, and cold showers. Potable water can be obtained from the picnic area.

Leave the recreation area behind, and soon reach FR 105. Cross the road and continue north in longleaf pines and turkey oaks. Abruptly turn right and cross a small creek on another plank bridge. Beyond this are interpretive signs identifying prevalent trees of the forest. Parallel a stream, then dive left into a titi thicket, emerging back to a wetland of bay, grass, and pine. The full name for bay is sweet bay magnolia. It grows primarily in wet areas. Its thick green leaves, with the silvery underside, are evident from afar on a windy day.

Leave the low, wet area and climb a hill to pick up a jeep track at 10.8 miles. Drop down to yet another wet area of bay, Atlantic white cedar, and cypress. Atlantic white cedar is an interesting tree. It is a tall evergreen with a spire-like crown and slender branches, and grows in a 50–100 mile belt along the coastline from Maine to Mississippi. This evergreen likes to grow in wet, swampy areas and alongside cool, clear waterways. During the Revolutionary War the wood of this tree was made into charcoal for gunpowder.

Stay alongside a wet area, looking for more Atlantic white cedars— the trail is in turkey oaks and pines. Reach a trail junction at mile 11.8. To your right, the blue-blazed Trail of Lakes leaves right and heads south to intersect the FT near Bonnet Lake. The orange-blazed FT turns left and enters a titi thicket. Keep along a cool, shady, elevated jeep trail. Climb out of the thicket onto Memery Island—an island of rich soil encircled by titi thickets and poorer, sandy soils. On top of the Memery are live oak, laurel oak, and magnolia. Peak out on the island at mile

12.1. Drop down again and cross a small creek, as the FT works around mud holes in the jeep trail.

At mile 12.7, leave the jeep trail. The savannas begin here. These savannas are mostly grass, but have scattered longleaf pines and cypress. Submerged during wetter times of the year, and fire-prone during drier times, these savannas harbor unique flora such as the pitcher plant. Butterworts and sundews are other carnivorous plants. Wildflowers are abundant here during the spring. The trailbed of thick grass is apt to be wet and clumpy. A swamp strand interrupts the savanna at mile 13.1. The grassy plains offer long views. At mile 14.0, cross another swamp strand, but soon return to the savanna, reaching FR 150 at mile 14.5.

Turn right on FR 150 and follow it a short distance to turn right on a lesser-used, often muddy jeep trail. Leave the jeep trail at mile 14.7, veering left as a footpath into a tall longleaf forest. The path is well blazed here, though the trailbed is indistinct. Emerge into a savanna at 15.2 miles. To the right of the trail is private land planted thickly in pines. Bisect a cypress slough at 15.5 miles, before walking through one last savanna and coming to SR 12 in Estiffanulga at 15.8 miles. This is the end of the FT in the Apalachicola National Forest.

## Florida Trail, Apalachicola National Forest Trail Log

### MEDART TO BRADWELL BAY

| | | |
|---|---|---|
| 0.0 | 66.4 | Leave Medart trailhead on US 319 |
| 0.3 | 66.1 | Traverse long and winding boardwalk through wooded wetland |
| 1.0 | 65.4 | Cross FR 356 |
| 1.4 | 65.0 | Reach longleaf-pine plantation |
| 1.9 | 64.5 | Cross stream on plank bridge in titi thicket, enter low hills broken by thickets |
| 3.9 | 62.5 | Step over blackwater stream, FT turns left |
| 4.7 | 61.7 | Stand of turkey oak atop a hill |
| 5.3 | 61.1 | Cross FR 321 |
| 5.5 | 60.9 | Cross FR 321-C, pass under power line, then cross stream on FR 321-C |
| 6.6 | 59.8 | Reach mature pineland after passing through pine plantation |
| 7.2 | 59.2 | Pass through area of many live oaks |
| 8.1 | 58.3 | Cross FR 365, drop down to banks of Sopchoppy River |
| 8.6 | 57.8 | Join FR 346 to cross Sopchoppy River on road bridge, return to woods |

## Florida Trail, Apalachicola National Forest Trail Log
### *(continued)*

| | | |
|---|---|---|
| **9.1** | **57.3** | Cross small creek on plank bridge after power line |
| **9.4** | **57.0** | Return to banks of Sopchoppy River, undulate along scenic river bluff |
| **10.1** | **56.3** | Leave river and climb onto pine flatwoods |
| **10.9** | **55.5** | Span Monkey Creek on footbridge |
| **11.4** | **55.0** | Step over small perennial stream after returning to Sopchoppy River |
| **12.4** | **54.0** | Step over another perennial stream, then circumvent wide swamp |
| **12.5** | **53.9** | Reach Sopchoppy River backcountry campsite after boardwalk bridges and before FR 329 |
| **12.7** | **53.7** | Reach Bradwell Bay Wilderness trailhead after turning left and walking on FR 329, trailside parking, enter Bradwell Bay Wilderness |

### BRADWELL BAY TO PORTER LAKE

| | | |
|---|---|---|
| **13.5** | **52.9** | Reach pine woods after crossing brush plain |
| **13.7** | **52.7** | FT spans small creek on remnants of road bridge |
| **14.1** | **52.3** | Enter palmetto-gallberry plain with blackened pine trunks |
| **14.7** | **51.7** | Stand of live oaks on trail-left, potential camping area, leave roadbed and turn left |
| **15.8** | **50.6** | Enter titi thicket to cross wide stream—no footbridge |
| **16.6** | **49.8** | Swing to south of saucer-shaped depression |
| **17.3** | **49.1** | Pass small pond |
| **17.6** | **48.8** | Intersect blue-blazed side trail leading left to FR 329 |
| **18.7** | **47.7** | Cross feeder stream of Monkey Creek in titi thicket |
| **19.1** | **47.3** | Ford Monkey Creek at site of bridge, may be bridge in future |
| **19.8** | **46.6** | Pass through swamp after sharp right turn |
| **20.0** | **46.4** | Intersect blue-blazed side trail leading left to FR 329, enter major swamp |
| **21.7** | **44.7** | Emerge onto pine island, last dry ground for miles, enter long swamp |
| **22.9** | **43.5** | Still waters—can be mucky, open, and deep |
| **23.9** | **42.5** | Enter area with thin swamp hardwoods, pass through one more deep section before picking up logging tram with canal on both sides of it |
| **25.2** | **41.2** | FT follows tram road as it veers right |
| **25.8** | **40.6** | Reach FR 314 and leave wilderness, FT turns right on FR 314 |
| **26.4** | **40.0** | Leave left from forest road into wet pine plantation |
| **27.4** | **39.0** | FT reaches non-numbered forest road to reach FR 388, turn right and follow FR 388 |

## Florida Trail, Apalachicola National Forest Trail Log
### (continued)

| | | |
|---|---|---|
| **28.3** | **38.1** | Leave forest road on left and enter pine plantation |
| **28.8** | **37.6** | Cross blackwater creek in titi thicket |
| **29.5** | **36.9** | Emerge onto SR 375, turn right and follow road over Smith Creek |
| **30.7** | **35.7** | Turn left onto Forest Highway 13 |
| **31.9** | **34.5** | Meet FT as it meets road from private land walkable only by Florida Trail Association members, cross Ocklockonee River on road bridge |
| **32.5** | **33.9** | Drop off road to enter primitive Porter Lake campground, pump well water, trailside parking |

### FLORIDA TRAIL ASSOCIATION MEMBERS ONLY

| | | |
|---|---|---|
| **29.5** | **36.9** | Emerge onto SR 375, turn right and follow road over Smith Creek |
| **30.2** | **36.2** | Turn left onto private land, follow FT through private land for 0.9 miles |
| **31.1** | **35.3** | FT meets road from private land walkable only by Florida Trail Association members, cross Ocklockonee River on road bridge |
| **31.7** | **34.7** | Drop off road to enter primitive Porter Lake campground, pump well water, trailside parking |

### PORTER LAKE TO VILAS

| | | |
|---|---|---|
| **32.5** | **33.9** | Leave Porter Lake Campground on foot trail, passing trail registration |
| **33.2** | **33.2** | Cross Forest Highway 13, soon span small branch on footlog |
| **34.2** | **32.2** | Span another small stream on a footlog, enter longleaf pine–wiregrass forest |
| **34.5** | **31.9** | Cross another stream on footlog |
| **35.5** | **30.9** | Cross FR 142 and span Hickory Branch on road bridge |
| **35.8** | **30.6** | Cross Coxes Branch on unusual suspension bridge, big pines around |
| **36.1** | **30.3** | Reach Jewell Tower backcountry campsite along Indian Creek |
| **36.2** | **30.2** | Cross CR 67 and Indian Creek on road bridge, enter hilly area |
| **37.7** | **28.7** | Cross FR 117 in turkey oak and longleaf pine |
| **38.5** | **27.9** | Reach FR 107, turn left on 107 only dry land for miles |
| **39.4** | **27.0** | Reach road junction with FR 126, FT keeps forward on 107 |
| **40.8** | **25.6** | FT leaves road left, into thick brush and pine, cross stream on plank bridge |

## Florida Trail, Apalachicola National Forest Trail Log
### (continued)

| | | |
|---|---|---|
| **42.1** | **24.3** | Reach spur trail leading right to Saplin Head backcountry campsite after crossing FR 175, FT keeps forward along headwaters of Bay Creek |
| **42.5** | **23.9** | Pick up jeep trail and step over Bay Creek, enter remote area, alternating between wiregrass prairie and floodplain swamps |
| **46.0** | **20.4** | Cross FR 107-B, stay in wiregrass and swamp |
| **47.7** | **18.7** | Bisect Saplin Head Swamp, turn north into wiregrass, turkey oaks, and longleaf pines |
| **48.5** | **17.9** | Reach FR 107 and span Black Creek on road bridge |
| **49.2** | **17.2** | Leave right from FR 107 after crossing tributary of Black Creek |
| **50.4** | **16.0** | Reach Vilas backcountry campsite beneath tall pines |
| **50.6** | **15.8** | Join FR 120, crossing Apalachicola Northern railroad tracks, leave road |

### VILAS TO ESTIFFANULGA

| | | |
|---|---|---|
| **50.9** | **15.5** | Reach SR 65, turn left, spanning New River on road bridge |
| **51.3** | **15.1** | Turn right onto FR 112, then leave road after passing through cattle guard, paralleling New River |
| **52.4** | **14.0** | Drop down along New River beneath cypress, ascend to pine plantation |
| **53.7** | **12.7** | Reach FR 112, cross Hostage Branch on road bridge, leave road |
| **54.8** | **11.6** | Descend into full-blown swamp, beware of slippery cut-log steps |
| **56.1** | **10.3** | Pass through private land, then join little-used FR 108-D |
| **56.8** | **9.6** | Cross FR 108, keep forward taking right fork, FR 108-E |
| **57.2** | **9.2** | Trail junction, Trail of Lakes comes in from right, Bonnet Pond is dead ahead, potential camping, FT turns left along shore of pond |
| **58.3** | **8.1** | Circle a normally dry lake bed, then pick up straight dug path |
| **58.7** | **7.7** | Reach FR 105, turn left, bridging Big Gully Creek, soon leave road left |
| **59.6** | **6.8** | Cross unnamed stream in titi thicket on plank bridge |
| **60.5** | **5.9** | Spur trail leads left to Camel Lake Recreation Area, camping, fishing, cold showers, and water available from picnic area, soon cross FR 105 |
| **61.4** | **5.0** | Pick up jeep track, stay alongside wet area |
| **62.4** | **4.0** | Trail of Lakes leaves right toward Bonnet Pond, FT turns left and climbs |
| **62.7** | **3.7** | Top out on Memery Island |

## Florida Trail, Apalachicola National Forest Trail Log
### (continued)

| | | |
|---|---|---|
| **63.3** | **3.1** | Leave jeep track, enter savannas broken by swamp strands |
| **65.1** | **1.3** | Reach FR 150, turn right and follow it short distance |
| **0.0** | | Reach SR 12 at Estiffanulga after passing in and out of savannas, end of FT in Apalachicola National Forest, roadside parking |

## Apalachicola National Forest Trail Information

Apalachicola National Forest
www.southernregion.fs.fed.us/florida

Apalachicola Ranger District
P.O. Box 579
Bristol, Florida 32321
(850) 643-2282

Wakulla Ranger District
1773 Crawfordville Highway
Crawfordville, Florida 32327
(850) 926-3561

# FOOTHILLS TRAIL

The Foothills Trail may be the most unsung, under-used, and underrated long trail in the Southeast. It traverses the Cherokee Foothills of the Southern Appalachians in North and South Carolina, through state parks, national forests, and state-owned preserves. In these lands are high ridgelines, wild and scenic rivers, deep rock gorges, wilderness areas, mountain lakes, clear trout streams, towering forests, and a number of incredible waterfalls stretching from one end of the path to the other. There are so many cascades along the Foothills Trail that I wonder why they didn't name it the Waterfall Trail.

The Foothills Trail is in full maturity. It is well marked, well maintained, and makes an excellent extended trek with ample camping opportunities. Several decades back, locals recognized the sheer number of natural resources found on the North Carolina–South Carolina border, and realized a path connecting these resources would be a great way to both enjoy and protect them. No one knows who exactly started the idea, but several persons and agencies converged to begin a "Foothills Trail." The first miles were laid out in Sumter National Forest back in 1968. (I actually met a former forest employee who was part of this effort.) As time passed, more agencies got involved, culminating with Duke Power Company laying out much of the heart of the trail. Duke Power has since sold their lands to the two states.

The Foothills Trail, extending 76 miles from Oconee State Park to Table Rock State Park, was completed in 1981. Over the years it has been fine-tuned. No doubt, you will notice the carefully built wood steps, waterbars, and bridges allowing hikers to traverse rugged areas throughout the trail. Since then, an alternative spur of the Foothills Trail has been extended along the Blue Ridge of South Carolina to reach Jones Gap State Park, making for a total of 86 miles. This extension, used as the Foothills Trail terminus in this guidebook, not only stays on the Palmetto State's rooftop, but also travels the Mountain Bridge Wilderness Area in Jones Gap and Caesars Head State Parks, enhancing and lengthening an already fantastic long trail. Of course, upstate South Carolinians, border North Carolinians, and Foothills Trail volunteers know full well the merits of this path. And after your hike, you too will give this Foothills Trail the recognition it deserves.

The southwest terminus of the Foothills Trail lies at Oconee State Park. Established in 1935, this mountain haven offers a campground that makes an excellent jumping off point. From here, the Foothills Trail starts its journey on ridgelines of pine and oak before descending to the Chattooga, a National Wild and Scenic River. The watercourse in this federally protected corridor, which forms the border between South Carolina and Georgia, froths and foams over rocky rapids, over named and unnamed waterfalls, and eventually slows to form large pools for swimming or fishing. For several miles, the Foothills Trail makes its way through the gorge cut by the Chattooga, where giant hemlock trees stand tall above incredible thickets of rhododendron. In places, the path lies directly alongside the Chattooga in wooded flats. Elsewhere, it works its way along precipitous bluffs.

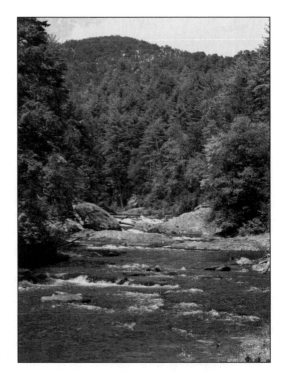

Chattooga River

The trail leaves the Chattooga and climbs Medlin Mountain, strad-dling the border of the Ellicott Rock Wilderness, before dipping down to East Fork Chattooga River, another mountain river replete with water-falls and wild trout. From here, the Foothills Trail traces Chattooga Ridge into North Carolina and the Nantahala National Forest, before descending into the Whitewater River Gorge. The Whitewater River really lives up to its name when it drops hundreds of feet into a gorge as Whitewater Falls. So does the trail. The river continues dashing and crashing among cabin-sized boulders back into South Carolina. The trail stays every bit as rugged as the gorge, then finally levels out in "The Hemlocks," a stand of evergreens. Nearby is a side path leading to an old-growth forest along Coon Branch and another trail leading to Lower Whitewater Falls.

The Foothills Trail leaves Whitewater Gorge and heads north, back into the Tar Heel State to enter an area known as the Jocassee Gorges. Several rivers and streams cut deep swaths in the mountains as they con-verge on Lake Jocassee, a clear impoundment rimmed in ridges. First, the Foothills Trail works down to the Thompson River, then east through remote lands to Bearcamp Creek and its premier destination, Hilliard Falls. Next comes the Horsepasture River. The Foothills Trail climbs over Bear Gap to Bear Creek, then to the Toxaway River and an area known as Cane Brake. Lake Jocassee adds another watery element to the event. Should hikers want to access the trail here, they will need to hire a boat shuttle—the only way in except by foot.

The trail next spans the Toxaway River, using the longest bridge of the entire trail. Then comes a challenging surprise known as "The Cat Stairs." Here, the path circles Lake Jocassee and ascends an ultra-steep path over a narrow ridge to Rock Creek, then reaches South Carolina once again. More remote lands lie between Rock Creek and Laurel Fork Creek. Naturally, hikers are greeted in the Laurel Fork Creek valley by a precipitous waterfall. The Foothills Trail then makes its way up the once-settled valley to a second falls, Double Falls. Ups and downs characterize the path as it skirts the south side of Flatrock Mountain. Then comes the big climb up to Sassafras Mountain, at 3,554 feet, the highest point in South Carolina.

The Foothills Trail diverges atop Sassafras. The white-blazed Foothills Trail heads south to its traditional ending at Table Rock State

Park, whereas the blue-blazed Foothills Spur Trail, fast becoming the preferred path, courses along the high ridge forming the divide between the two Carolinas. The ups and downs along this section are very challenging, though it eases up once it reaches an historic woods road built by the Civilian Conservation Corps during the Great Depression of the 1930s. A real sense of remoteness falls upon the path. Next, the Foothills Trail enters the Mountain Bridge Wilderness Area, which encompasses parts of Caesars Head State Park and Jones Gap State Park. Walk along the very edge of the Blue Ridge, then descend into the Middle Saluda River watershed. It should come as no surprise that waterfalls are an ongoing feature here. The Foothills Trail makes its way down this valley tracing an historic toll road built in the 1850s, then comes to an end at Jones Gap State Park headquarters.

Overnight camping opportunities are numerous, with some restrictions. Backcountry camping is prohibited in Oconee and Caesars Head State Parks and the Whitewater River Gorge. (Whitewater River Gorge is an especially attractive area where the namesake natural resource is tightly protected.) Backcountry camping within the Sumter National Forest is by permit only, except in the Chattooga River corridor and Ellicott Rock Wilderness, where you don't need one. The permit system in Sumter doesn't restrict campers to specific sites. Backcountry camping at Jones Gap State Park is by permit only and restricted to specific sites.

Generally, most camping occurs along streams, though some high-country camping can be done. Water is generally accessible throughout the trail. Angling is a very viable option here. And with so much water, hiking the Foothills Trail is a year-round proposition, though summer can be very hot; you will want to be near water as often as possible. The area around Lake Jocassee can be busy with boaters on summer weekends. Spring offers an abundance of wildflowers in the many lush valleys. My most enjoyable moments have been in fall, with the vibrant colors and cooler temperatures. Winter can be variable, with snow in the high country and entire days below freezing a very real possibility, though milder days occur with regularity.

In keeping with the tradition of the Appalachian Trail and all the other trails in this guidebook, the Foothills Trail is described heading south to north, though in this case it is more southwest to northeast. This generally keeps the afternoon sun at your back, making for a cooler hiking experience. Backpackers can extend their end-to-end trek from a week to two weeks or more, if they are willing to bring all their supplies with them, as I have before. Be apprised that access to stores and post offices along the trail is virtually nonexistent. This is due to the remoteness of the trail and the nearly continuous wild lands it traverses, which is ultimately the preferred situation. Road crossings are frequent enough to cache supplies in a car or have others meet you, though the trail passes through a 30-plus mile section without easy road access. Hiking the Foothills Trail end-to-end was one of my most enjoyable outdoor experiences. Hopefully it will be for you, too.

## Foothills Trail, Oconee State Park to Burrells Ford

| | |
|---|---|
| **Length:** | 16.4 miles |
| **Trail Condition:** | Excellent |
| **Highs:** | Chattooga Wild and Scenic River, some views, Big Bend Falls, Kings Creek Falls |
| **Lows:** | Limited camping first 8 miles |
| **Season:** | Year-round; lowlands away from water can be uncomfortably hot in summer |
| **Difficulty:** | Moderate, lots of short ups and downs |
| **Use:** | Heavy near Chattooga River, moderate elsewhere |
| **Tips:** | Consider car camping at Oconee State Park and getting an early start the next day in order to make it to camp at Chattooga River watershed. |
| **Campsites:** | 8.0, 10.9, 11.9, and 14.4 miles |

**OCONEE STATE PARK TRAILHEAD:** From Walhalla, South Carolina, drive north on South Carolina 28 north for 8.5 miles to SC 107. Turn right on SC 107 and follow it 2.5 miles to the state park, on your right. From here, follow the signs through the park to the Foothills Trail, on the road to cabins 7–13.
**BURRELLS FORD TRAILHEAD:** From Walhalla, South Carolina, drive north on SC 28 for 8.5 miles to SC 107. Turn right on SC 107 and

follow it for 8.9 miles to gravel FR 708. Turn left on FR 708 and descend for 3 miles. Burrells Ford parking area will be on your left. The Foothills Trail crosses FR 708 just before reaching the parking area.

This most southwestern section of the Foothills Trail starts at one of South Carolina's oldest state parks, a destination in its own right. Oconee State Park makes for a good jumping off point, whether you stay in the campground, with full amenities, or go upscale with one of their rental cabins. The Foothills Trail begins in piney woods near Stratton Mountain. Leave Stratton Mountain for Long Mountain, which offers views from its steep slopes, before dropping to the superlatively attractive Chattooga River. However, the trail doesn't stay beside the river for long, as it climbs over a knob on a river bend. Make your way along Rock Gorge before returning to the Chattooga's edge. At times, the trail comes so close to the water that it is nearly in the river, passing through wooded flats and over small side streams with that everywhere-you-look beauty. Leave the Chattooga again in the vicinity of Round Top, only to drop down once more to the river near Big Bend Falls, a surging force of water pinched between the walls of the gorge. Beyond here, the trail stays fairly close to the Chattooga, until it enters the Kings Creek Valley. Here, a side trail leads a short piece to the "must see" Kings Creek Falls. Beyond Kings Creek, the trail pulls away from the Chattooga to soon reach the Burrells Ford parking area. Burrells Ford is a walk-in camping area that used to have auto access until the Chattooga was designated as "Wild and Scenic" in 1974. This designation restricted auto access.

Camping, fishing, and wildlife viewing opportunities are numerous along the Chattooga. However, no camping is allowed outside of the campground in Oconee State Park. The section of the Sumter National Forest outside the Chattooga requires a free permit, which can be obtained by calling (864) 638-9568. Please call two weeks in advance. There are no suitable camping sites until 8 miles in, near Sumter's Lick Log Creek. Level campsites with water are located a 8.0, 10.9, 11.9, and 14.4 miles.

❀    ❀    ❀

The white-blazed Foothills Trail starts inauspiciously near the Oconee State Park cabins. The trail begins across from the parking area and runs in conjunction with the Hidden Falls Trail for the first mile or so. Be sure to register at the self-registration board near the parking area. Enter the pine-oak woods, and at 0.4 miles, reach the junction with the Tamassee Knob Trail, which leads right 1.6 miles to Tamassee Knob. Veer left here and work around the headwaters of Horse Bone Branch to make the south end of Long Mountain. Leave the state park and enter the Sumter National Forest at mile 1.2, then intersect a closed road. Keep forward here as the Hidden Falls Trail leaves right. At mile 2.0, a side trail leaves left for the Long Mountain fire tower. The tower is closed to the public, but the peak does offer wintertime views. Beyond this, other views are open to the east before the Foothills Trail dips over to the west side of Long Mountain and works its way down toward Clear Branch, then over a couple of wooden bridges down the narrow upper reaches of Tamassee Creek. Head away from the creek up a steep hollow. Once out of the hollow, views open to the southeast. The trail reaches SC 107 at mile 4.6. Do not cross the road; instead, stay right and immediately re-enter the woods, heading up a timber road. Soon, veer off the timber road in piney woods and work around the east slope of Dodge Mountain. Views open through the trees to your right. Bisect an old logging road at mile 5.5, then turn left away from the ridgeline, reaching gravel Cheohee Road at mile 5.9. Cross the road at an angle, soon reaching SC 107 at mile 6.0.

Cross SC 107, and circle around the south end of Chattooga Ridge, picking up a streamlet feeding Lick Log Creek in woods of tall white pine. Turn north, paralleling Lick Log Creek below. Span a bridge at mile 6.8 and reach a junction. A side trail leads left 200 yards to the Thrift Lake parking area. Span another small branch before reaching the Nicholson Ford parking area at mile 7.5. Keep descending, now along noisy Pigpen Branch, to reach a camping spot in a grove of white pine at mile 8.0. Immediately span Lick Log Creek on a footbridge, then pass more camping areas to span Lick Log Creek again. Make a short but steep descent to reach an important trail junction at mile 8.3.

You have now entered the Chattooga Wild and Scenic River corridor, the boundary of which is marked with light-blue blazes. Here, the dark-blue-blazed Chattooga Trail leads left to cross Lick Log Creek just below Lick Log Falls, a short distance away, then heads downstream along the Chattooga. The Foothills Trail, now running in conjunction with the upstream-bound portion of the Chattooga Trail, leads right. It follows beside the edge the Chattooga River Gorge on a rocky, rooty path alongside rock bluffs, ranging far above the audible Chattooga. Top out at mile 8.7. Trace an old woods road through hickories and oaks, cutting over a knob that the river works around. Pass huge hemlock trees as you descend to make the Chattooga at mile 10.1. The wild and scenic river froths and crashes over rocks, then gathers in pools, building steam before continuing its tortured journey downstream. It is unusual to see rivers of this size be federally designated as Wild and Scenic in the East. A streamside flat offers campsites, especially near Simms Field. A riverside beach and large swimming hole marks Simms Field, which is reached just after a footbridge at mile 10.9.

After Simms Field, the trail stays along the river, so close that at times the path may be submerged when the water is up. Reach another beach across from a rock bluff at mile 11.3. The trail soon leaves the river and works around Round Knob on a steep mountainside before intersecting a side trail to Big Bend Falls at mile 12.8. This rough, unmarked side path heads left, dipping below a rock house to reach the upper part of the huge, crashing Big Bend Falls. The Foothills Trail follows switchbacks away from the river before descending past Fraser magnolias and rock formations to once again near the river at mile 13.1. Short side trails lead to the water. The trail crosses an eroded roadbed at an angle and passes the small falls of a feeder branch just before reaching a trail junction at mile 13.6. Here, the Big Bend Trail leads right 2.7 miles to Cherry Hill campground.

The Foothills/Chattooga Trail forges ahead, bridging a small branch above a 6-foot cascade. Drop alongside the Chattooga River, rock-hopping upstream at the water's edge. Look around and try to grasp the absolute beauty of this river. During times of high water, look to the right for a rough, high-water route that circumvents this section. Keep upstream and make a flat with camping possibilities on a riverbend at mile 14.4. Switchback up the side of the gorge in heavy rhododendron among rock outcrops, then turn into the King Creek watershed, picking up an old wagon road to reach a trail junction at mile 15.3. A spur trail continues forward to reach Burrells Ford Walk-in Campground, but keep with the white blazes as the path veers uphill to the right to reach another junction at mile 15.7. Here, another spur trail leaves right 0.2 miles to King Creek Falls: Don't bypass this waterfall's 80-foot drop into a clear pool. The trail heads back downstream to span Kings Creek, then climbs away from the stream to meet Burrells Ford Road (FR 807) at mile 16.4. Just before the road, a spur trail leads forward to make the Burrells Ford parking area. The Foothills Trail turns right, to cross FR 807, and heads for Medlin Mountain.

## Foothills Trail, Burrells Ford to Bad Creek Access

| | |
|---|---|
| **Length:** | 14.6 miles |
| **Trail Condition:** | Good |
| **Highs:** | Ellicott Rock Wilderness, Whitewater River Gorge, waterfalls, some views |
| **Lows:** | Rough, slow trail between NC 281 and Whitewater Gorge |
| **Season:** | Year-round, summer is tolerable on higher ridges and in gorge |
| **Difficulty:** | Moderate to difficult |
| **Use:** | Moderate; heavy on warm weekends in Whitewater River Gorge |
| **Tips:** | Very limited camping, be prepared to adjust your daily hiking mileage |
| **Campsites:** | 6.9 and 9.7 miles |

**BURRELLS FORD TRAILHEAD:** From Walhalla, South Carolina, drive north on SC 28 for 8.5 miles to SC 107. Turn right on SC 107 and follow it for 8.9 miles to gravel FR 708. Turn right on FR 708 and descend for 3 miles. Burrells Ford parking area will be on your left. The Foothills Trail crosses FR 708 just before reaching the parking area.

**BAD CREEK ACCESS TRAILHEAD:** From the junction of SC 11 and SC 130 just north of Salem, South Carolina, head north on SC 130, South Bruce Rochester Memorial Highway. Keep north for 10.2 miles to the gated entrance of the Bad Creek Project. Drive up to the gate and it

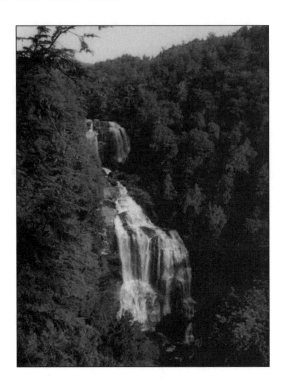

Whitewater Falls

will open (from 6 a.m. to 6 p.m.) Pass through the gate and keep down-hill for 2 miles and turn left at the sign for the Foothills Trail, driving 0.3 miles to a large parking area. The Bad Creek Access Trail starts in the far left-hand corner of the parking area.

This slice of the Foothills Trail is composed of several diverse landscapes. Leave Burrells Ford and ascend Medlin Mountain on the edge of the Elli-cott Rock Wilderness. The Medlin Mountain section of the Foothills Trail is part of an excellent loop within the Ellicott Wilderness, so it can be somewhat busy. Crest Medlin Mountain and descend into the rugged East Fork Chattooga River Valley, with its waterfalls choked in dense woods and rhododendron, to meet SC 107. Here, trail traffic slackens considerably as the trail crosses quiet Chattooga Ridge and enters North Carolina near Round Mountain, which offers good high-country camp-ing. Work around the side of Grassy Knob and gain views before toiling on a rough path to reach Whitewater Gorge. Your entrance begins with the roar of Whitewater Falls, then gets even more raucous deep in the gorge, with its rugged array of big boulders, cascades, and tall trees. The trail winds along the steep sides of the gorge before opening up in "The Hemlocks," a shady wooded flat where a homesite once stood. Here, a side trail leads right, to the Bad Creek Access, as well as an old growth forest along Coon Branch.

Campsites with water are limited to a small flat near SC 107 on East Fork Chattooga and on the old Foothills Trail near Round Mountain. No camping is allowed in Whitewater Gorge. However, there is a designated campsite on the Foothills Trail 0.6 miles beyond the lower end of Whitewater Gorge and the Bad Creek Access Trail. Along this section, camping flats with water are located at 6.9 and 9.7 miles.

❀    ❀    ❀

The Foothills Trail/Chattooga Trail leaves Burrells Ford Road (FR 807) just uproad from the dead end parking area. Switchback up through a dry forest to meet a small stream above a low-flow, 40-foot waterfall over a rockface at 0.4 miles. Grab water here and keep climbing to a trail junction at 0.6 miles. Here, the Foothills and Chattooga trails part ways. The Chattooga Trail leaves left, going a mile to the Chattooga River; the Foothills Trail ascends right, up the nose of Medlin Mountain in hickory, pine, and mountain laurel. Soon, come alongside the border of Ellicott Rock Wilderness, as marked by signs on trail-left. The trail winds upward, in and out of small hollows, then makes three wide switchbacks to crest out at mile 2.2. Swing around a knob, then regain the crest, only to circle around two more knobs, breaking the 3,000 foot elevation mark as it crosses Chattooga Ridge. Drift downward to reach Fish Hatchery Road at mile 3.9.

Cross the gravel Fish Hatchery Road to head northeast into the woods on a narrow single-track path coursing beneath a hillside of mountain laurel. Step over a spring branch at mile 4.5, and soon enjoy views of Fork Mountain through the trees to the northwest. Split a gap at mile 5.7, then descend toward East Fork Chattooga River, crossing several streamlets. Pass under a small power line at mile 6.3, then reach a pretty, four-tier waterfall above a footbridge. The East Fork soon comes into view and features a wide cascade and deep pool of its own. Walk a bit more, passing a second waterfall and reach a rough side trail descending to this fall. At mile 6.9, look left into a potential camping flat intertwined in rhododendron. Beyond this, the Foothills Trail turns away from the East Fork to ascend an intermittent streambed, then crosses a flowing streamlet to reach SC 107 at mile 7.2. Dead ahead is the Sloan Bridge Picnic Area. The Foothills Trail turns right, away from the picnic area, to cross SC 107. The path becomes much less used at this point, since most day hikers take the Fork Mountain Trail, which starts beyond the picnic area, to head west toward Ellicott Rock, the point where Georgia, South Carolina, and North Carolina meet.

Past SC 107, the trail moderately but steadily ascends the side of Chattooga Ridge, with Jacks Creek, a feeder branch of the East Fork, audible below and to the left. Mountain laurel and rhododendron crowd the path. Reach the crest of Chattooga Ridge and an old woods road at mile 8.3. Here, the mountainside drops sharply to the southeast—look for a side path leading right to a decent view. At mile 8.6, reach the North Carolina state line and enter the Nantahala National Forest. Circle around to the south side of Round Mountain on a rough path, making a gap and a trail junction at mile 9.7. This trail, the old Foothills Trail, leads left 0.3 miles down to a camping area in maple and birch near a perennial stream. A few other sites lie across the flowing stream, then left, up along the stream. The current Foothills Trail continues forward, heading for the gap to Grassy Knob, shifting to the southeast side of the knob and gaining views to the southeast amid sassafras, hickory, and chestnut oak. Switchback downhill, criss-crossing a streamlet entangled in mountain laurel, then make an eastward tack to reach NC 281 at mile 11.9. Keep forward and cross the paved road. The Foothills Trail resumes at the back end of the dirt parking area on the far side of the road. Descend on an old, wide roadbed fronted by wooden vehicle barriers. This area was once a picnic area, as evidenced by the concrete foundations for two outhouses to the left of the path.

The Foothills Trail leaves the old roadbed and creeps down along the declivitous lower reaches of Grassy Knob to span a small stream on a footbridge. The path is narrow and rocky and the going is slow before reaching a side trail leading left to the Whitewater Falls parking area at mile 12.3. Keep forward, walking amid large boulders, from the parking area, before meeting the side trail to Whitewater Falls Overlook. Ascending the 111 steps to the observation area is absolutely worth the time. The main trail curves right and begins to switchback via more steps into the depths of the Whitewater Gorge. (Remember, no camping is allowed in the gorge.) The roar of the river is audible, but the water can't be seen until mile 12.9. Giant boulders clog the river as the water loudly forces its way downstream. An iron suspension bridge allows you to cross and adds a great watery view. Once across the bridge, notice remnant anchor supports of an old bridge that was washed away by the powerful water. Head downstream and shortly span Corbin Creek on a smaller bridge. Look upstream in the cool, dark valley for a tall waterfall above more boulders.

The going gets slow again as the trail scales the side of the valley via steps and bridges to reach a wooded flat and the South Carolina state line at mile 13.5. Soon, leave the flat to twist around a rockface before spanning Pams Creek on a footbridge at mile 14.0. A flat opens here and the Foothills Trail enters "The Hemlocks." Stroll along and look for piled boulders in this former farmland. Reach a major trail junction at mile 14.6. To the right, across a bridge over the Whitewater River, is the Bad Creek Access Trail, which leads 0.6 miles to the parking area described in the directions above. The Coon Branch Trail begins across the same bridge, leading left through an old growth forest. The Foothills Trail continues to the left, reaching a designated campsite 0.6 miles distant. Also this way is the trail to Lower Whitewater Falls.

# Foothills Trail, Bad Creek Access to Rocky Bottom

| | |
|---|---|
| **Length:** | 30.3 miles |
| **Trail Condition:** | Good |
| **Highs:** | Jocassee Gorges, numerous waterfalls, Lake Jocassee, fishing possibilities |
| **Lows:** | Boat noise at Lake Jocassee on summer weekends, many wood steps awkward for backpackers |
| **Season:** | Year-round; best during spring, early summer and fall. Low elevation makes for hot hiking in summer |
| **Difficulty:** | Moderate to difficult, numerous ascents and descents in gorges |
| **Use:** | Generally moderate, heavy near Lake Jocassee |
| **Tips:** | Plan for 30 miles without road access; consider using a private boat shuttle available midway on this section |
| **Campsites:** | 0.6, 2.7, 3.9, 4.8, 5.9, 8.6, 11.2, 17.0, 18.3, 22.9, 25.5, 26.3, and 27.5 miles |

**BAD CREEK ACCESS TRAILHEAD:** From the junction of SC 11 and SC 130 just north of Salem, South Carolina, head north on SC 130, South Bruce Rochester Memorial Highway. Keep north for 10.2 miles to the gated entrance of the Bad Creek Project. Drive up to the gate and it will open (from 6 a.m. to 6 p.m.) Pass through the gate and keep downhill for 2 miles and turn left at the sign for the Foothills Trail and drive 0.3 miles to a large parking area. The Bad Creek Access Trail starts in the far left-hand corner of the parking area.

**ROCKY BOTTOM TRAILHEAD:** At the junction of SC 11 and US 178, 9 miles north of Pickens, South Carolina, take US 178 north for 8.1 miles to Rocky Bottom. Just after US 176 spans Rocky Bottom Creek on a bridge, turn left onto a gravel road and drive 0.3 miles to the Laurel Valley parking area.

This is one long and spectacular section of trail. It is hard to find 30 miles of trail in the East without crossing a major road, but the Foothills Trail delivers. It occasionally passes by normally gated gravel roads on state lands, but hikers can't count on finding them in the maze of gravel roads or on finding them open. Leave the lower Whitewater Gorge to pass the side trail to Lower Whitewater Falls, then travel east into an area known as the Jocassee Gorges. The remote Thompson River is the first beautiful body of water visited. Next, meander through piney woods and reach Bearcamp Creek, which has good camping and a waterfall. Keep east to reach Horsepasture River. Climb away from that gorge, winding through low hills to find quiet Bear Creek. More hilltopping leads to an area known as Cane Brake and Lake Jocassee. Here, the Toxaway River flows beneath the longest suspension bridge on the entire trail. This is where a boat shuttle can divide this section. Next come the surprisingly tough Cat Stairs and pretty Rock Creek. Twist and turn amid a labyrinth of old timber roads to reach Laurel Fork Creek, which has waterfalls and good campsites. Make an easy walk up this valley before again hitting a rough section in hill country to reach Rocky Bottom trailhead. Duke Power once owned these lands and built much of the trail here, which has many bridges and steps. They have since sold their land to North and South Carolina.

Savor this slice of the Foothills Trail. The numerous creeks and rivers will entice you to camp along them, not only for the natural beauty and good campsites, but also for the trout and smallmouth-bass fishing. The potential for a boat shuttle adds a planning twist for section trail-trompers. For a boat shuttle, contact Hoyett's Grocery in Salem, South Carolina, at (864) 944-9016. If you like solitude, try to hit the Lake Jocassee area midweek and not during high summer. Campsites with water are located at 0.6, 2.7, 3.9, 4.8, 5.9, 8.6, 11.2, 17.0, 18.3, 22.9, 25.5, 26.3, and 27.5 miles.

❁   ❁   ❁

Begin this section at the junction of Bad Creek Access Trail and the Foothills Trail at the bottom of Whitewater Gorge, 0.6 miles from the Bad Creek Access parking area. Leave the Whitewater River, ascending along a tiny feeder stream on the edge of former farmland. The path becomes steep and meets an old logging road and a trail junction at 0.5 miles. The Lower Whitewater Falls Trail leads forward 0.9 miles to an overlook of the lower falls. The Foothills Trail continues left along wooded hills to reach a second junction at 0.6 miles. To your right, down a hill, is a decent designated campsite with a fire grill in a flat. A tiny spring flows from a bluff adjacent to the camp.

Keep north in oak woods, then descend into a rhododendron-filled draw. The trail begins a pattern of picking up old timber roads then leaving them on single-track paths, sometimes in dry oak-hickory woods and sometimes in rhododendron-filled hollows. While the single-track sections are easy to follow, keep an eye open for the white blazes of the Foothils Trail when on timber roads, and don't walk too far without seeing a blaze. Boundary blazes on the trees mark reentry into North Carolina.

Begin an extended descent to reach the Thompson River at mile 2.7. The trail turns downriver a short distance, then comes to a flat beside a trail bridge and a riverside campsite, which oozes isolation. Span the long bridge over the Thompson to find a second campsite, then rise from the gorge along a small branch, using steps and switchbacks to meet a timber road. At mile 3.3, reach a junction. To the right, an old woods road leads toward Musterground Road. The Foothills Trail stays left, passing a tiny stream dripping over a rockface on trail-left. Ascend past this and note another old road leading right as the trail curves left at mile 3.9. Down this old road is a designated, but crummy, campsite on a slope; it may or may not be signed. Water can be had back at the previous tiny stream.

The trail soon dives into a hollow, taking many steps downward, bridges another tiny stream twice, and emerges onto a dirt road. On the road, descend past posts from a metal gate to reach a bridge spanning Bearcamp Creek at a downward angle at mile 4.8. The streamside is thick with hemlock and rhododendron. Just ahead is the short, 0.3-mile spur trail to Hilliard Falls. Take this trail to find a tall cascade dripping over a rockface; the water drops a good 60 feet into a surprisingly large pool. A campsite lies near the falls as well as on the trail just beyond the trail junction.

The Foothills Trail follows Bearcamp Creek downstream amid a carpet of partridgeberry, crossing the creek on another footbridge and undulating along the side of the valley before crossing a third bridge to enter an appealing camping flat at mile 5.9. Here, the trail picks up an old roadbed and turns right, downstream on Bearcamp Creek, passing another campsite. Eventually, work away from the watercourse, which is still audible as it drops to Lake Jocassee. At mile 6.5, the trail makes a sharp left turn and the sounds of water disappear. Follow a timber road around the south side of Narrow Rock Ridge. The shiny rocks on the ground, which look like broken glass, are mica. The wide path makes for easy walking in and out of hollows, until, out of nowhere, the trail heads left, up a series of steps and away from the timber road at mile 8.4. The Horsepasture River becomes audible as the path ascends, then descends alongside a cabin-sized boulder and a small rock house to reach the Horsepasture River and a small campsite at mile 8.6.

Cruise across the Horsepasture River on a 115-foot bridge, but be sure to look upstream at the big, bouldery watercourse. Ascend 103 steps, then keep climbing on a dirt trail to reach a logging road and climb more. Leave the logging road, and span a couple of small ravines to reach an elaborate suspension bridge over another ravine at mile 9.7. The trail then meets another logging road and winds through a stand of pines, which offers a southwest view beyond the trees. Drop down to reach Bear Gap and a four-way junction of old logging roads. Leave left and pass around a metal gate to reach Bear Creek at mile 11.2, where you'll find an inviting campsite beneath hemlocks.

Span Bear Creek on a wooden footbridge and swing around a wide flat, ascending to a gap with a power line at mile 11.9. Enter Gorges State Park and drop down to cross Cobb Creek on a footbridge with a handrail at mile 13.2. Ascend the nose of a piney ridge, jumping on and off an eroded timber road. Begin working down toward Lake Jocassee among old timber roads on Grindstone Mountain. Keep an eye peeled for the white blazes, which show the way across a perennial stream on a small bridge at mile 15.1. Climb a bit past the stream then begin the 1-mile descent to Cane Brake, reaching Lake Jocassee at mile 16.4. A trail sign-board indicates a lake access point, where a boat shuttle could drop off hikers.

The Foothills Trail swings north, following the Toxaway River arm of Lake Jocassee, hopping on and off an old timber road. Make a surprising climb on steps around a steep bluff before dropping to the 225-foot-long suspension bridge over the Toxaway River. This span, at mile 17.0, offers a fine view of the river. Soon cross Toxaway Creek on a smaller bridge, then enter a large and popular camping flat—at 1,170 feet, the lowest point on the entire Foothills Trail. Cruise through the flat and head south along the lakeshore, passing the rock remnants of an old homesite. Just ahead are the Cat Stairs. Suddenly, climb too many steps up an ultra-steep knob to reach a resting bench. The "Steps from Hell" continue to reach the ridgeline and an old woods road with good lake views. Descend very steeply on more steps and wonder if Duke Power must have gotten a bad quarterly report when they built this section. More steps lead off the ridgeline to mercifully make Rock Creek at mile 18.3. Span a footbridge to reach an attractive, shaded campsite in a large flat. A side trail leads a short piece downstream along Rock Creek to meet Lake Jocassee.

Skirt the lake beyond Rock Creek and enjoy watery views. Also note more rock piles indicating old farmland. Pass one last lake access point before turning away from the water. Rise sharply on a maze of logging roads and single-track paths, eventually re-entering South Carolina. Leave a single-track path at mile 19.1 and turn left onto a very wide former woods road with a broken forest canopy. Drift through an open gap and reach a metal gate at mile 20.2. The trail veers right off the road and parallels a closed access road in young pine woods. Cross the closed access road to reach a second metal gate at mile 20.9. Keep forward to drop off the ridgeline and walk beneath a younger moist forest with many tulip trees and vines. Reach a trail junction at mile 22.2. Here, a side trail leads right to a boat access on the Laurel Fork Creek arm of Lake Jocassee. Turn left and bridge Jackies Branch, leaving Lake Jocassee for good.

The trail passes through an obvious old road cut before reaching an overlook of Laurel Fork Falls at mile 22.7. This steep falls is a froth of white that seems to emit more water than is possible once you see Laurel Fork Creek. Keep forward on an old roadbed and reach a trail junction at mile 22.9. Here a side trail leads right to a suspension bridge spanning Laurel Fork Creek, reaching a good campsite and former homesite. The Foothills Trail forges ahead, passing around a metal gate, then crossing a footbridge at mile 23.5. Turn left into this part-time auto access area and keep upstream, passing a newer road bridge. Re-enter full-fledged forest in rich woods thick with galax and doghobble, then cross another footbridge at mile 23.8. The trail hops off and on an old road that has been closed since the area was bought by the state in the late 1990s. Farther upstream, the trail uses old wooden road bridges to span the creek. At other times, it parallels the old road in woods. At mile 25.5, the trail spans Laurel Fork Creek on a footbridge, enters a camping flat, and immediately turns left to span Laurel Fork again on a footbridge. Here the Foothills Trail and old road part ways: the old road heads to Laurel Fork Gap while the single-track path leads just a short distance to Double Falls. A spur trail leads to the base of the two-tiered, low-flow fall.

Climb stairs around the falls as the Laurel Fork Creek valley pinches in and the woods thicken. Span several footbridges as the trail switches from side to side as it follows the narrowing stream, pinched in by rock bluffs. One of these footbridges is an old log that has had handrails placed on it. At mile 26.3, the trail abruptly turns right to leave Laurel Fork Creek, the last easily accessible water for several miles. A campsite lies just across the stream. The going becomes slow and rough as the trail works its way out of the watershed on single-track and timber roads. Drop down to reach a slightly sloped designated camping area at mile 27.5. The camp is in a hardwood forest with a very small stream just beyond it.

The Foothills Trail then keeps east along the south slope of Flatrock Mountain, winding in and out of dry hollows beside rock bluffs. Pass a side trail, leading right, to a rock outcrop and winter views at mile 28.7. Soon descend sharply. A gravel road becomes visible to your right. Come near the road once before a final short climb, then take wooden steps down to the Laurel Valley Access parking area at mile 30.3, the end of this section. The Foothills Trail continues left, down the gravel road to shortly reach US 178 and Rocky Bottom.

# Foothills Trail, Rocky Bottom to Jones Gap State Park

| | |
|---|---|
| **Length:** | 24.4 miles |
| **Trail Condition:** | Good |
| **Highs:** | Highest point in South Carolina, historic toll road, Mountain Bridge Wilderness Area, waterfalls, views |
| **Lows:** | Limited water, some walking along little-used gravel road |
| **Season:** | Year-round; best during late spring, early summer, and fall |
| **Difficulty:** | Strenuous |
| **Use:** | Moderate, heavy on weekends at Jones Gap State Park |
| **Tips:** | Keep apprised of water supply as first 14 miles have limited water |
| **Campsites:** | 1.6, 4.1, 7.2, 9.1, 11.5, 11.9, 12.2, 19.7, 22.3, and 24.4 miles |

**ROCKY BOTTOM TRAILHEAD:** At the junction of SC 11 and US 178, 9 miles north of Pickens, South Carolina, take US 178 north for 8.1 miles to Rocky Bottom. Just after US 176 spans Rocky Bottom Creek on a bridge, turn left onto a gravel road and drive 0.3 miles to the Laurel Valley parking area.

**JONES GAP STATE PARK TRAILHEAD:** From Pickens, South Carolina, take SC 8 north for 15 miles to SC 11. Veer right onto SC 11 and follow it 2 miles to US 276. Turn right on US 276 and follow it 4 miles to River Falls Road. Turn left on River Falls Road, and keep forward for 5.5 miles as it turns into Jones Gap Road to dead end at Jones Gap State Park.

This challenging and long parcel of the Foothills Trail offers many rewards to those who traverse it. Leave Rocky Bottom and begin the ascent of Sassafras Mountain, highest point in South Carolina. Pass by a large rock house to reach Chimneytop Gap. Keep climbing to make

Sassafras Mountain and some views. Here, the Foothills Trail splits. The traditional route leaves south for Table Rock State Park, 9 miles distant. The alternative route, which this guidebook follows, stays in the high country, tracing the North Carolina–South Carolina state line along the Blue Ridge. It makes challenging ups and downs, crossing the historic Emory Gap Toll Road to meet another historic gravel road built in the 1930s by the Civilian Conservation Corps. The state line ridge here oozes solitude and offers the best views on the entire Foothills Trail. Top out on pine-studded Slicking Mountain and leave the state line at Gum Gap, then enter Mountain Bridge Wilderness Area, which encompasses portions of South Carolina's Caesars Head and Jones Gap State Parks. Descend into the perched Matthews Creek valley, nearing Raven Cliff Falls. Gain views from very edge of the Blue Ridge before descending into the Middle Saluda River watershed, which some argue to be the most beautiful in the Palmetto State. (They will get no argument from me.) Pass more waterfalls along an historic toll road built in the 1850s before reaching trail's end at Jones Gap State Park.

Campsites are limited here, by terrain and regulations. It's all high-country camping with limited water until the Mountain Bridge Wilderness, where backcountry camping is prohibited at Caesars Head State Park and allowed by permit only at Jones Gap State Park. Numerous designated sites are located along the Middle Saluda River, though you must get a permit in advance to camp at these sites. Permits can be obtained at either Caesars Head or Jones Gap State Parks before your trip or by making a 1-mile road walk to the Caesars Head park office. Furthermore, since the trail straddles the Carolina state lines past Sassafras Mountain, the south side of the trail is off limits to camping, as it is part of the City of Greenville watershed. Camping on this section is easier than the above information suggests. All it takes is some planning. Also, keep apprised of water availability. Look for potential campsites with water at 1.6, 4.1, 7.2, 9.1, 11.5, 11.9, 12.2, 19.7, 22.3, and 24.4 miles. The last campsite is at trail's end.

❋   ❋   ❋

The Foothills Trail leaves the Laurel Valley parking area and descends on the gravel parking lot access road to reach US 178 and Rocky Bottom

Creek at 0.3 miles. Turn right and span the road bridge, then immediately enter woods to the left. Climb sharply away from US 178 up a moist ravine to make a small knob at 0.7 miles. Surprisingly, descend before resuming the climb, passing a large rock house at 1.0 mile, uphill on trail-left. Keep ascending while working around Chimneytop, bridging three streambeds along the way. At mile 1.6, after the third small bridge, look right for a flat on an old roadbed that serves as a campsite. The nearby spring branch may be nearly dry in fall. Ascend by steps up a rockface and circle around a ridgeline that offers views, then reach a wide woods road and drift into Chimneytop Gap at mile 2.1. Immediately cross F. Van Clayton Highway, a quiet road that leads to Sassafras Mountain.

From the highway, head uphill in woods, passing by an old logging road cut in a second-growth hardwood forest rife with tulip trees. At mile 2.6, climb some steps around a rockface and keep ascending to reach a side trail leading left to Balancing Rock. This overlook avails far-reaching views to the southwest, including Lake Jocassee. Now, swing around to the north side of the mountain and pass through a gap to emerge on the south side of the mountain at White Pine Point, where the trail picks up a woods road. White pines were planted here after the old-growth forest was harvested in 1971. Reach an open gap at mile 3.9 and turn right. Just as you begin to wonder about the rest of the climb, the trail leaves the road left at mile 4.1, following some wooden steps up, then up some more. If you keep going forward on the roadbed, it leads to a campsite and a miniscule spring branch. Be apprised F. Van Clayton Highway is fairly close, so close that the trail crosses the road again at mile 4.3. Walk along the highway a bit then look left, crossing the road to make the final ascent up Sassafras Mountain. Just before reaching the top, look for a side trail leading left to a view to the west. Shortly there-after emerge onto the mountaintop at mile 4.7, where a clearing, site of a former tower, sits at 3,554 feet.

Follow a ragged paved road down from the mountaintop. Just before reaching a metal gate, look left for a wide, blue-blazed trail head-ing into thick woods. This is the Foothills Spur Trail, which stays in the high country and extends the hike. The traditional white-blazed Foothills Trail keeps forward past the gate, then leads left into the woods and winds 8.8 miles to its terminus at Table Rock State Park.

To continue on the Foothills Spur Trail, follow the blue blazes past a small cell tower and a benchmark. The red blazes to the right of the trail mark the Greenville watershed boundary. The path narrows and drops off the steep slope of Sassafras Mountain, straddling the state line. You will also see state-line boundary markers. Turn off the main ridgeline to reach steep and narrow Sassafras Gap at mile 5.8. Look both ways from this gap. You are standing on the Emory Gap Toll Road, which once crossed the mountains from Pickens County in South Carolina to Transylvania County in North Carolina. If you are in need of water, head a rough 0.3 miles north into North Carolina.

From the gap, the Foothills Trail makes a tough ascent toward Whiteoak Mountain in a forest of maple, oak, and mountain laurel. A view can be had just to the left of the trail at mile 6.1. Keep ascending steeply to make a woods road at mile 6.4. Undulate on the ridgeline over Whiteoak Mountain, leaving the woods road. At mile 7.1, the trail makes a sharp 90° left turn, then descends to come very near a dirt road to your left at mile 7.2. Just ahead, in a pine grove, is a nice campsite. Water can be had by leaving left on the foot trail from camp to reach the dirt road. Walk a few feet left on the dirt road to an intersection. Turn right and enter a semi-permanent hunt camp. A clear reliable spring is to the left of the camp.

The Foothills Trail ascends, then exits beside the dirt road at mile 7.5. Turn sharply right, back into the woods. Continue in remote country along the state line, ascending toward Big Spring Mountain, passing over a couple of knobs, topping out on Big Spring Mountain at mile 7.8. Descend very steeply, skip over a second knob, then dive more steeply down a rhododendron-hemlock ravine into a kudzu-covered forest. Reach a woods road, turn right, and take it a short distance to a gap at mile 8.8. Turn left away from the road and climb insanely upward to top out on a knob. Drop to a logging road and a roadside campsite at mile 9.1. To the right of the grassy campsite is a trail leading to a small creek. Head up the rock and gravel road, portions of which were built in the 1930s by the Civilian Conservation Corps. As the road curves left at mile 9.7, the trail leaves right on a single-track path into the woods, which may catch you off guard. Ascend, passing a side trail leading to a big rockface. Pop back out on the road and keep uphill on Dolves Mountain.

Pass an open rock outcrop on the left at mile 10.2. You can see far to the north, across the East Fork French Broad River Valley and the mountains of the Nantahala National Forest. This is the best view on the entire Foothills Trail.

Follow switchbacks downhill, making an extended descent along the north slope of Bursted Rock Mountain to reach a low point at mile 11.5. Here, the road forks. To the left is a stream that just passes under a culvert on the road and a possible campsite, your last camping-with-water opportunity before reaching Jones Gap State Park. Take the right fork and climb along the state line. Drop back down after a sharp right turn, and at mile 11.9, look left for a seldom-used campsite in a hollow. Just beyond it is a small spring with hard-to-get water. The road veers right again and drops to reach Slicking Gap on a left curve at mile 12.2. Another seldom-used campsite and difficult spring are to the left.

Soon, reach an obvious road split. Veer right, uphill, and begin climbing Slicking Mountain. Reach a bench of the mountain and level off, then make the final jump, reaching the top of the pine-cloaked mountain at mile 13.1. The canopy is open overhead, and at 3,200 feet the walking is easy. Pass around a metal gate at mile 13.3, and descend a sometimes-eroded road to reach Gum Gap at mile 13.9. Here, the trail turns right, leaving the state line, and passes around a metal gate to enter the Mountain Bridge Wilderness Area. At this point, the Foothills Trail runs in conjunction with the Gum Gap Trail as it descends the perched Matthews Creek valley, an elevated valley atop a mountain. Moderately descend on a wide roadbed accompanied by pine trees and granite outcrops. Step over a feeder branch of Julian Creek at mile 14.2. Keep downhill along Julian Creek to a junction at mile 14.8. The trail continues forward while another woods road crosses Julian Creek on a decrepit wooden bridge. Descend the attractive valley and reach Matthews Creek at mile 15.4. Rock-hop the clear mountain stream. Look for Matthews Creek cascading off to your right through the trees. Pass around a gate at mile 15.8 and keep forward. Pass through a junction of woods roads to reach a trail intersection at mile 16.1. Here, the Naturaland Trust Trail leaves right 0.4 miles to a platform overlooking Raven Cliff Falls.

Now, the FST leaves left, up an eroded roadbed, then down to cross a feeder stream of Matthews Creek flowing through a culvert at mile 16.8. Ascend a rocky trailbed amid dense vegetation and reach another trail junction at mile 17.3. Here the trail leaves right, passes around a metal gate, and leads toward the edge of the Blue Ridge. Climb steeply around a knob, then come to yet another junction near a rain shelter at mile 17.7. Here, the Raven Cliff Falls Trail heads 0.7 miles to a viewpoint of the falls. The Foothills Trail turns left, now running in conjunction with the Raven Cliff Falls Trail toward US 276. Head east, running along the escarpment of the Blue Ridge, descending to step over an intermittent streambed then go up some steps. Just past these steps, at mile 18.1, look right for a side trail leading to an outcrop and view of the Matthews Creek watershed and beyond. Occasional views open up as the trail keeps east, then turns left to cross an old dam and a drained lake that is now a wetland. Climb away from the dam to reach US 276 at mile 19.0. If you haven't gotten a permit to backcountry camp at Jones Gap State Park, you can walk 1 mile south, right, to the Caesars Head office to get a permit.

The Foothills Trail crosses the road. Look in the left corner of the parking area below for the Tom Miller Trail. The Coldspring Branch Trail leaves the right hand corner of the lot. Take the Tom Miller Trail, which runs in conjunction with the Foothills Trail. Dip into a rich forest, jump over a small knob, then descend steeply down the nose of a rib ridge to reach a thick dark forest and the Middle Saluda River at mile 19.7. Three backcountry campsites are in the vicinity here. Turn right and head downstream to meet the Jones Gap Trail, with which the Foothills Trail runs in conjunction. The Jones Gap Trail traces an old toll road built in the 1850s by Solomon Jones. Span the Middle Saluda on a log bridge at mile 20.0, as the Saluda falls far below you. The trail enters a section known as "The Winds," as in wind a clock, for the way the trail switchbacks back and forth. Two ultra-attractive waterfalls lie at the base of "The Winds." Continue downstream and pass a large rock house.

The Foothills Trail now stays far above the Middle Saluda for a good distance. Pass a couple more campsites and feeder streams of the Middle Saluda flowing off the Blue Ridge. The path makes its way near the river again and a trail junction at mile 22.3. The Coldspring Branch Trail leaves right to make US 276 in 2.6 miles. The Foothills Trail stays near the Middle Saluda as it continues to form scenic unnamed waterfalls and pools. This area has many designated campsites. Some sections of the trail are wet, as small seeps cross the Foothills Trail while flowing to the main river. Make a sharp right turn and leave the old toll road to span the Middle Saluda at mile 23.4. Across the bridge, the Ishi Trail heads uphill to meet the Rim of the Gap Trail. The Foothills Trail keeps downstream on a rocky section as the valley opens up. Intersect the Rim of the Gap Trail just before crossing a wide bridge over the Middle Saluda and reaching Jones Gap State Park headquarters at mile 24.4, where you'll find a pay phone, parking, and information. The park offers walk-in tent camping sites in addition to the backcountry campsites. To reach the parking area, keep downstream, passing the old fish-hatchery pond, and take a small path back over the river to your car.

## Foothills Trail Log

### OCONEE STATE PARK TO BURRELLS FORD

| | | |
|---|---|---|
| 0.0 | 85.7 | Foothills Trail leaves Oconee State Park |
| 0.4 | 85.3 | Trail junction, Tamassee Knob Trail leaves right, trail leaves left |
| 1.2 | 84.5 | Leave Oconee State Park, enter Sumter National Forest |
| 2.0 | 83.7 | Side trail leaves left for Long Mountain fire tower (no view) |
| 4.6 | 81.1 | Trail comes alongside SC 107. Do not cross road |
| 5.9 | 79.8 | Reach gravel Cheohee Road |
| 6.0 | 79.7 | Cross paved SC 107, descend into Chattooga River valley |
| 6.8 | 78.9 | Side trail leaves left 200 yards to Thrift Lake parking area |
| 7.5 | 78.2 | Reach Nicholson Ford parking area |
| 8.0 | 77.7 | Pigpen Branch, campsites, descend to enter Chattooga Wild and Scenic River corridor |
| 8.3 | 77.4 | Trail junction, Foothills Trail turns right, runs conjunctively with Chattooga Trail |
| 8.7 | 77.0 | Top out on knob as Chattooga River flows around knob |
| 10.1 | 75.6 | Reach Chattooga River, campsites |
| 10.9 | 74.8 | Simms Field, beach area, campsites |
| 12.8 | 72.9 | Unsigned and rough side trail leads left to Big Bend Falls |
| 13.6. | 72.1 | Trail junction, Big Bend Trail leads right to Cherry Hill Campground, Foothills Trail descends toward Chattooga River |
| 14.4 | 71.3 | Trail turns right at river bend, campsite, ascend away from Chattooga |
| 15.3 | 70.4 | Trail junction, side trail leads left to Burrells Ford Walk-in Campground, Foothills Trail veers right, uphill |
| 15.7 | 70.0 | Side trail leads right 0.2 miles to King Creek Falls, trail spans Kings Creek |

## Foothills Trail Log *(continued)*

| | | |
|---|---|---|
| **16.4** | **69.3** | Spur trail keeps forward to reach Burrells Ford campground parking area. Trail turns right to reach FR 807, Burrells Ford Road. Cross FR 807 |

### BURRELLS FORD TO BAD CREEK ACCESS

| | | |
|---|---|---|
| **16.8** | **68.9** | Reach small stream with waterfall. Last water source for 4 miles. |
| **17.0** | **68.7** | Trail junction, Foothills and Chattooga trails split. Keep right, uphill and ascend Medlin Mountain, coming along border of Ellicott Rock Wilderness |
| **18.6** | **67.1** | Crest out on Medlin Mountain |
| **20.3.** | **65.4** | Cross Fish Hatchery Road |
| **20.9** | **64.8** | Step over spring branch, work toward East Fork Chattooga River |
| **22.7** | **63.0** | Pass under small power line then reach four-tier waterfall above footbridge |
| **23.3** | **62.4** | Campsite along East Fork Chattooga in flat below, to left of trail |
| **23.6** | **62.1** | Cross SC 107 at Sloan Bridge Picnic Area, ascend Chattooga Ridge |
| **24.7** | **61.0** | Crest out on Chattooga Ridge, views to southeast |
| **25.0** | **60.7** | Reach North Carolina state line, enter Nantahala National Forest |
| **26.1** | **59.6** | Reach gap between Round Mountain and Grassy Knob. Campsites 0.3 miles down gap. Trail keeps right around south slope of Grassy Knob |
| **28.3** | **57.4** | Cross NC 281 |
| **28.7** | **57.0** | Side trail leads left to Whitewater Falls parking area, soon reach side trail leading left to Whitewater Falls viewing platform, descend into Whitewater Gorge |
| **29.3** | **56.4** | Span Whitewater River on iron suspension bridge, descend along gorge |
| **29.9** | **55.8** | Enter South Carolina, keep descending |
| **30.4** | **55.3** | Span Pams Creek on footbridge, soon enter "The Hemlocks" |
| **31.0** | **54.7** | Trail junction, Bad Creek Access Trail leaves right 0.6 miles to parking. Trail turns left away from Whitewater River |

### BAD CREEK ACCESS TO ROCKY BOTTOM

| | | |
|---|---|---|
| **54.2** | **31.5** | Lower Whitewater Falls Trail keeps forward, trail turns left |
| **54.1** | **31.6** | Side trail leads right to designated campsite with spring |
| **33.7** | **52.0** | Cross Thompson River on long bridge, riverside campsites |
| **34.3** | **51.3** | Trail junction. Foothills Trail leaves left, side trail leads right toward Musterground Road |

## Foothills Trail Log *(continued)*

| | | |
|---|---|---|
| **34.9** | **50.8** | Side trail leads right to crummy designated campsite, weak spring fairly near |
| **35.8** | **49.9** | Span Bearcamp Creek, campsite, side trail leaves left 0.3 miles to Hilliard Falls |
| **36.9** | **48.8** | Span Bearcamp Creek for third time, campsites, pick up jeep road |
| **37.5** | **48.2** | Trail makes sharp left while working around Narrow Rock Ridge |
| **39.4** | **46.3** | Trail leaves jeep road, ascends and descends steps |
| **39.6** | **46.1** | Span Horsepasture River on 115-foot bridge, small campsite nearby |
| **40.7** | **45.0** | Elaborate suspension bridge over dry ravine |
| **42.5** | **43.2** | Bear Creek, campsite in flat beneath hemlocks |
| **42.7** | **43.0** | Reach gap at power line and enter Gorges State Park |
| **44.0** | **41.7** | Span Cobb Creek on footbridge, ascend nose of piney ridge |
| **45.9** | **39.8** | Cross small perennial stream on footbridge, descend to Lake Jocassee |
| **47.4** | **38.3** | Reach Lake Jocassee at Cane Brake, potential boat shuttle access point. Swing around Toxaway River arm of Lake Jocassee |
| **48.0** | **37.7** | Cross Toxaway River on 225-foot suspension bridge, soon span Toxaway Creek on footbridge and reach large camping area |
| **49.3** | **36.4** | Reach Rock Creek with good camping and lake access after making "Cat Stairs." Leave lake area for Laurel Fork Creek |
| **51.2** | **34.5** | Pass first of two metal gates |
| **53.2** | **32.5** | Trail junction, side trail leads right 0.3 miles to Lake Jocassee, Foothills Trail turns up Laurel Fork Creek Valley, leaving Lake Jocassee area for good |
| **53.7** | **32.0** | Overlook of Laurel Fork Falls |
| **53.9** | **31.8** | Side trail leads right to designated campsite along Laurel Fork, Foothills Trail keeps upstream, crossing Laurel Fork on bridges |
| **56.5** | **29.2** | Span Laurel Fork on footbridge, enter camping flat and immediately cross creek again on footbridge. Just ahead is Double Falls, valley pinches in |
| **57.3** | **28.4** | Trail abruptly leaves Laurel Fork Creek, last campsite on Laurel Fork across creek |
| **58.5** | **27.2** | Designated campsite in flat with very small stream just beyond |
| **59.7** | **26.0** | Side trail leads right to outcrop and winter view |
| **61.3** | **24.4** | Take wood steps down to Laurel Valley Access parking area |

## ROCKY BOTTOM TO JONES GAP STATE PARK

| | | |
|---|---|---|
| **61.6** | **24.1** | Cross Rocky Bottom Creek and US 178, begin ascent of Sassafras Mountain |

## Foothills Trail Log *(continued)*

| | | |
|---|---|---|
| 62.3 | 23.4 | Large rock house uphill to left of trail |
| 62.9 | 22.8 | Camping flat to right of trail on far side of tiny spring |
| 63.4 | 22.3 | Cross F. Van Clayton Highway at Chimneytop Gap |
| 63.9 | 21.8 | Side trail leads left to view at Balancing Rock |
| 65.2 | 20.5 | Reach open gap after Pine Point, turn right on woods road |
| 65.4 | 20.3 | Trail leaves roadbed left, ahead is small campsite on roadbed with minuscule spring nearby |
| 65.6 | 20.1 | Trail crosses F. Van Clayton Highway, make final ascent up Sassafras Mountain |
| 66.0 | 19.7 | Reach top of Sassafras Mountain, highest point in SC at 3,554 feet, descend, then look left for blue-blazed Foothills Spur Trail re-entering woods on wide roadbed |
| 67.1 | 18.6 | Reach Sassafras Gap after big descent, Emory Gap Toll Road crossed here |
| 67.4 | 18.3 | View to left of trail, ascend over Whiteoak Mountain |
| 68.5 | 17.2 | Campsite in white pine grove just after trail nears a dirt road. Water is on trail leading left from campsite, then left on dirt road, then right at dirt road intersection by semi-permanent hunt camp. Cruise along NC-SC state line |
| 70.4 | 15.3 | Emerge onto wide gravel road at campsite. Small creek downhill to right. Keep uphill on gravel road |
| 71.0 | 14.7 | Trail leaves road right, re-enters woods. Keep uphill on Dolves Mountain |
| 71.5 | 14.2 | Great view to north of East Fork French Broad valley after resuming gravel road |
| 72.8 | 12.9 | Reach low point at fork in road. Take upper fork. Water just below lower fork. Look from here forward for the next mile for camping |
| 73.2 | 12.5 | Little-used campsite in hollow to left. Difficult spring nearby |
| 73.5 | 12.2 | Reach Slicking Gap on left turn. Campsite and difficult spring in hollow to left. Another road split, keep uphill |
| 74.4. | 11.3 | Reach top of Slicking Mountain. Soon pass around metal gate and descend |
| 75.2 | 10.5 | Reach Gum Gap. Turn right, descending into Mountain Bridge Wilderness Area |
| 76.1 | 9.6 | Trail junction. Foothills Trail keeps forward, side trail leads right across Julian Creek |
| 76.7 | 9.0 | Rock-hop Matthews Creek |
| 77.4 | 8.3 | Trail junction. Foothills Trail turns left and ascends |
| 78.6 | 7.1 | Trail turns right toward edge of Blue Ridge. Road keeps forward |
| 79.0 | 6.7 | Trail junction. Foothills Trail turns left, Raven Cliff Falls Trail keeps forward 0.7 miles to view |

## Foothills Trail Log *(continued)*

| | | |
|---|---|---|
| **80.3** | **5.4** | Reach US 276. Caesars Head ranger station is 1 mile right. Foothills Trail crosses US 276 and heads left, in conjunction with Tom Miller Trail |
| **81.0** | **4.7** | Reach Middle Saluda River and Jones Gap Trail. Turn right, run in conjunction with Jones Gap Trail down Middle Saluda River. Backcountry campsites in area |
| **81.3** | **4.4** | Span Middle Saluda on footbridge. Soon enter "The Winds" |
| **83.6** | **2.1** | Trail junction. Coldsprings Branch Trail leaves right. Foothills Trail keeps forward, soon passes more backcountry campsites |
| **84.7** | **1.0** | Span Middle Saluda on bridge. Ishi Trail leaves after bridge. Foothills Trail keeps downstream, enter rocky area |
| **85.7** | **0.0** | Cross bridge and reach Jones Gap State Park headquarters. Parking area is just downstream past fish hatchery and bridge |

## Foothills Trail Information

Foothills Trail Conference
P.O. Box 3041
Greenville, South Carolina 29602
www.foothillstrail.org

Sumter National Forest
www.fs.fed.us/r8/fms

Sumter National Forest
Andrew Pickens Ranger District
112 Andrew Pickens Circle
Mountain Rest, South Carolina
  29664
(864) 638-9568

Nantahala National Forest
www.cs.unca.edu/nfsnc/

Nantahala National Forest
Highlands Ranger District
2010 Flat Mountain Road
Highlands, North Carolina
(828) 526-3765

South Carolina State Parks
www.southcarolinaparks.com

Oconee State Park
624 State Park Road
Mountain Rest, South Carolina
  29664
(864) 638-5353

Table Rock State Park
158 East Ellison Lane
Pickens, South Carolina 29671
(864) 878-9813

Caesars Head State Park
8155 Geer Highway
Cleveland, South Carolina 29635
(864) 836-6115

Jones Gap State Park
303 Jones Gap Road
Marietta, South Carolina 29661
(864) 846-3647

# PINHOTI TRAIL

The master path of Alabama, the Pinhoti Trail (PT) is a National Recreation Trail that extends for over 100 miles along the southernmost extension of the Appalachian Mountains. Located in the Talladega National Forest, the trail passes through two wilderness areas (Dugger Mountain and Cheaha) as well as Cheaha State Park, the site of Alabama's highest point. Those who follow the Pinhoti will find piney ridges, rock outcrops with far-reaching views, richly wooded hollows, and quiet wooded lakes fed by clear streams both small and large.

Pinhoti is the Creek Indian word for "turkey home." You may or may not see some wild turkeys on your journey, among other critters such as deer, but you will see tracks. This hiker-only trail is blazed by white turkey tracks, either painted on trees or marked with metal diamonds emblazoned with turkey tracks. The standard blue painted blazes are also used from time to time. Hikers who visit this trail during hunting season will need to acquire camping permits, available from either district ranger station. This is to inform hikers of what type of hunting is going on where. Hikers doing the entire 104 miles will need to carry all their supplies with them, though at the approximate halfway point, hikers can make about a 2.5-mile side trek to Heflin to stock up.

The trail may be the pride of Alabama, but the state of Georgia claims its share of this trail. While the completed section of the trail stops just short of Georgia, the long-term plan is to extend the Pinhoti Trail through northwest Georgia, connecting to another long trail detailed in this book, the Benton MacKaye Trail. The Benton MacKaye Trail currently connects to the Appalachian Trail, thus a hiker could start in Alabama and hike all the way to Maine, or even beyond to Cape Gaspe in Quebec on the International Appalachian Trail! The Pinhoti Trail through Georgia is currently a work in progress, so Pinhoti thru-hikers in Georgia have a lot of road walking to reach the Benton MacKaye Trail.

❀   ❀   ❀

Starting at the trail's southern terminus near Porters Gap, the Pinhoti marches up the side of Talladega Mountain, only to drop steeply to Talladega Creek, crossing a railroad line to pass by a couple of houses, its most civilized point. Things quickly return wild as the path returns to the crest of Talladega Mountain, running the ridge on a rocky treadway. Water is scarce up here as the path keeps a northeasterly course, finally descending to water near Adams Gap. Once at Adams Gap, the path enters the Cheaha Wilderness, tracing Alabama's highest ridgeline, where rock outcrops offer stunning views of the wooded expanse beyond. Pass through Cheaha State Park, then descend to the Blue Mountain Backcountry Area, which is centered on the upper Hillabee Creek valley. In both the upper and lower valley, clear streams course though rich wooded hollows where beech and tulip trees grow straight and tall, bordered by hills of oak, pine, and hickory. Features like this 3,500-acre swath of wildness, where streams fall steeply to form attractive cascades, are what add variety to the Pinhoti. Pass near a different watery feature, Morgan Lake, before keeping north to cross US 431. This lesser-hiked section passes under I-20 near Heflin before emerging into the northern half of the national forest.

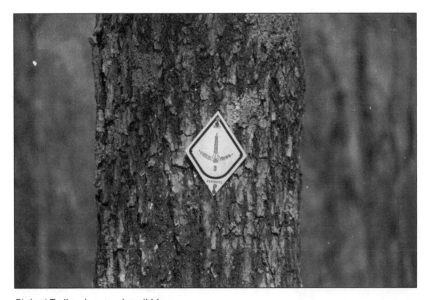

Pinhoti Trail turkey-track trail blaze

The Pinhoti enters the land of lakes and streams in the Shoal Creek watershed. The translucent waters of area creeks, broken by steep, wooded hills are the setting for bass-fishing opportunities and camping at two trail shelters. Some of these streams have been dammed, forming several quiet wooded lakes. These quiet lakes also offer fishing and diverse environments. More watery environments await in the Choccolocco Creek watershed. This watery portion of the Pinhoti contrasts with the trail's tail end. Here, the Pinhoti leaves hill and creek country to climb onto dry, rocky ridges and mountains, capped by a trek over Dugger Mountain, Alabama's second highest peak. Numerous challenging ascents and descents in lesser-traveled terrain lead to US 278 and the Pinhoti Trail's most northern public parking. Beyond here, the Pinhoti is being extended to the Georgia state line and beyond, but trailside parking is sketchy and the path disjointed. Stay tuned as the Pinhoti evolves.

# Pinhoti Trail, Porters Gap to Cheaha State Park

| | |
|---|---|
| **Length:** | 26.3 miles |
| **Trail Condition:** | Good |
| **Highs:** | Views, rock outcrops, Cheaha Wilderness |
| **Lows:** | Long dry sections of trail, very rocky path in places |
| **Season:** | Year-round; best during spring and fall, summer can be hot |
| **Difficulty:** | Moderate to difficult |
| **Use:** | Moderate, heavy in Cheaha Wilderness |
| **Tips:** | Start your hike with water and fill up wherever you can, especially in dry times |
| **Campsites:** | 5.1, 13.4, and 21.3 miles |

**PORTERS GAP TRAILHEAD:** From Exit 168 on I-20 east of Pell City, take AL 77 for 21.7 miles south to reach the Chandler Gap trailhead, which will be on the left.

**CHEAHA TRAILHEAD:** From Exit 191 on I-20 near Anniston, head south on US 431 for 3.6 miles to Cleburne County 131. A sign states "To Talladega Scenic Drive." Turn right on Cleburne County 131 and follow it 0.4 miles to Talladega Scenic Drive, AL 281. Turn left on the scenic drive, AL 281, and follow it 11.9 miles to the Cheaha trailhead, which will be on your left.

This beginning segment of trail follows the southernmost portion of the entire Appalachian Range. The Appalachian Range starts way up in Quebec and extends southwesterly through the eastern United States and eventually into Alabama. These mountains you will be walking are the very end of the range; go further south and the Appalachians drop off into wooded hills and the Gulf Coast Plain. The Porters Gap trailhead, your starting point, is the southern terminus of the entire Pinhoti Trail.

From Porters Gap, the path heads north along the ridgeline of Talladega Mountain, soon dropping to Talladega Creek. After crossing the creek and a railroad line, the path once again ascends Talladega Mountain, passing a small stream, your last water for miles, before resuming a northeasterly course along the very rocky north slope of the mountain. Drop to Clairmont Gap, only to climb again, crisscrossing the ridgetop, eventually descending to another perennial water source before climbing to Adams Gap. Enter the Cheaha Wilderness in a section ravaged by fire during the late 1990s. Walk in the north shadow of Talladega Mountain before making a steep and challenging climb to the ridgecrest, breaking the 2,000 foot elevation mark and keeping northeast along Alabama's most lofty ridge. This is a land of boulders and rock formations. Massive rocks protrude from the side of the mountain on a bluffline. These outcrops avail far-reaching views that will simply amaze, as verdant forests extend as far as the eye can see. This superlative beauty attracts crowds, so expect to have company on weekends. Keep along the ridgeline to enter Cheaha State Park and the end of this section.

Places to camp are fairly numerous in this section—water is not. You must plan your camping around obtaining water. Bring a water bag, fill up, and you will have far more camping options. There are no resupply points until reaching the state park, where you'll find a country store that sells picnic and convenience store–type items. The state park also has a lodge with a dining room, cabins, and a campground for a change of pace. Campsites with water are located at 5.1, 13.4, and 21.3 miles.

❁    ❁    ❁

Start your hike by leaving the Porters Gap trailhead, entering a pine-oak woodland and immediately coming to a trail sign. Begin walking a needle-covered single-track path heading toward Talladega Mountain. Soon pass an old jalopy at 0.3 miles, and ascend in and out of coves, crossing dry streambeds where hardwoods dominate overhead. Reach Chandler Gap at mile 1.4. Notice the old woods road slicing through the gap. The path now runs the rocky crest of the mountain under a broken canopy. The sunny conditions foster more blueberries, which ripen in early summer. At mile 2.1, switch around to the north side of the mountain, still climbing to pass a small rock shelter. The area offers obscured views to the north and south. Descend in fits and starts to reach paved CR 394 at mile 3.2. Turn left here, tracing the blacktop to cross the Seaboard Coast Railroad, then Talladega Creek on a road bridge. Pick up gravel FR 600-2, and follow it uphill, passing a junky area before ascending left into the woods at mile 3.5.

Work back up Talladega Mountain via switchbacks. Reach the crest, then criss-cross the ridgeline. At mile 4.8, bisect FR 600-2. Keep forward here on a footpath, avoiding the jeep road that veers downhill to the right. The trail descends to reach a perennial stream at mile 5.1. Notice the beech trees in this steep, moist hollow. Small campsites can be found downstream of the crossing or a few minutes beyond the crossing up on a ridgeline. This is the last reliable water for 8 miles, so fill your canteens. Climb away from the stream to level out in a boulder field offering expansive views to the south. Ascend to reach FR 600-2 at mile 6.0. Cross the gravel road and descend in rocky woods. The trail passes near a precipitous canyon-like drainage on trail-left before falling into a pattern of winding through moist drainages with intermittent streams broken by drier pine rib ridges. The trail here is very rocky, and summertime brush obscures the pathway; you will spend your time watching the ground nearly every step instead of enjoying the scenery.

By mile 8.5, the rockiness has abated as the trail passes underneath two power lines before arriving at Clairmont Gap. Cross the paved road splitting the gap and walk a few feet on FR 600-2, then climb left into the woods, once again ascending Talladega Mountain. Pass by some brushy woods that are recovering from fire, then head up several switchbacks to gain the ridgeline, where there are views of the Talladega Creek valley and the southern portion of Talladega Mountain. Wind along the ridge among rocks in open forest that is growing up in locust and black-berry. Come here between April and June and you may see an interesting wildflower—the fire pink. The pink refers not to the color (the flower is actually red) but to the shape of the lower petals, which appear to have been notched, or pinked, by scissors. Eventually settle in along the north side of the ridge, which makes for easier travel, passing below rock out-crops. Red maple is abundant in these woods. Cross FR 600-2 in a gap at mile 11.1, swinging around the south-facing slope of Burgess Point, where pines are more prevalent. Cross FR 600-2 again at mile 11.9, curving around a couple of high knobs. Descend rapidly beyond the two knobs, crossing little-used FR 6370 at mile 13.2. Continue descending, crossing a streambed six times. Reliable water can be found at the sixth crossing. Fill up here, whether camping near the stream or not. A few small campsites are in this steep watershed, but you may have to carry your water with you a bit. Climb over a low ridge away from the stream and step over a second small creek before ascending sharply toward Adams Gap, coming to a trail junction at mile 15.2. The Skyway Trail leads left 6 miles to Lake Chinnabee. The Pinhoti Trail leads right to reach Adams Gap and Talladega Scenic Drive at mile 15.3.

Cross the paved drive and head toward the descending gravel road. Turn left from the gravel road and climb into woods that were burned in a late 1998 arson fire. Soon, come to a trail signboard and enter the 7,400-acre Cheaha Wilderness, established in 1983. Sweetgum trees, with their star-shaped leaves and gumball-like seed pods, thrive here in the aftermath of the fire. These trees are pioneers, growing in disturbed areas, making shade for other less-sun-tolerant species. The trail soon lev-els off, hopscotching in and out of burned and unburned woods as it winds along the north slope of Talladega Mountain. Western views are common in burned areas as are dead trees fallen across the trail. At mile 16.5, step over a stream, leaving the drainage for sun-burnished former pine country. Other, more suspect streambeds beyond may or may not have water. Continue the pattern of moist hollows alternating with piney rib ridges.

At mile 18.8, come to an abrupt, signed right turn. The Pinhoti picks up an old jeep track and begins climbing toward the main ridgeline. The trail rises along the mountain before leaving the woods road at a sharp left switchback at mile 19.1. Now, pick though an enormous boulder field as you follow the foot trail. The climbing begins in earnest, switch-backing among interesting rock formations, less appreciated because hikers are huffing and puffing at this juncture. Slice between a rock wall just before emerging onto level ground at mile 19.7. A side trail leads right to a bluff that offers far-reaching westward vistas. Keep ascending onto the ridgetop, eventually breaking the 2,000-foot barrier. Squeeze through boulders at mile 20.0. Look left for more views. Descend among mountain laurel to pass an intermittent stream. Sassafras, recognized by its hand- or mitt-shaped leaves, grows here in abundance. The roots of this small tree or bush are used to make tea and were once one of America's first exports, while America was under British rule.

Leave the intermittent stream and gain the western bluffline again, coming to other outcrops with fantastic views. Campsites become more frequent. Step over a year-round spring that disappears only in abnormally dry weather just before arriving at a trail junction at mile 21.3. The Chinnabee Silent Trail leaves left to Lake Chinnabee. The Odum Trail leads right 4 miles to High Falls. The Pinhoti continues forward beyond the popular camping area in a mixture of pine and hardwoods. Swing around the west side of Little Caney Head, regaining the crest at mile 21.9, then drift over to the western mountainside, where dramatic bluffs drop hundreds of feet and offer nearly continuous views. Open outcrops beckon hikers to stop and absorb the sights from Talladega Mountain, extending south toward the horizon and mile upon mile of forestland in the west.

Leave the bluffline and traverse rock fields before reaching a trail junction at mile 22.8. The Cave Creek Trail leaves right. The Pinhoti Trail veers left and struggles through a rugged boulder field. Temporarily leave the Cheaha Wilderness and the boulder field. The white outcrop of McDill Point is visible to the west. Descend to a cove, crossing a dry streambed at mile 23.8. Turn south and climb through pine woods, reaching a trail junction at mile 24.2. A side trail leads left 0.25 miles to the large McDill Point Overlook. The Pinhoti Trail descends past an odd, tall rock then climbs among gray rampart-like rock walls to soon emerge at another outcrop. Talladega Scenic Drive is visible below in this mountain and valley panorama. Views and outcrops continue until the Pinhoti turns away from the ridgeline and enters Cheaha State Park near a level gap, leaving the wilderness for good.

Trace the turkey tracks up toward Hernandez Peak, passing a granite plaque commemorating the Cheaha Wilderness. At mile 25.2, top out on Hernandez Peak in grassy woods. This is the highest ground on the entire Pinhoti Trail at 2,340 feet. Descend from this peak through a break in the bluffs to step over a streambed in a gap. A jeep trail parallels the Pinhoti as it picks up a lower bluff with more views. Step over the jeep trail and slip off the east side of the ridgeline, coming to a trail junction at mile 26.3. To your right, a side trail leads a short distance to the Cheaha parking area. The Pinhoti Trail continues forward, reaching Cleburne in 25.9 miles.

# Pinhoti Trail, Cheaha State Park to Cleburne

| | |
|---|---|
| **Length:** | 25.9 miles |
| **Trail Condition:** | Good |
| **Highs:** | Views, waterfalls, Blue Mountain Backcountry Area |
| **Lows:** | Major road crossings latter half |
| **Season:** | Year-round; best during spring and fall, summer can be hot |
| **Difficulty:** | Moderate to difficult |
| **Use:** | Heavy near state park, moderate to light elsewhere |
| **Tips:** | Try to avoid camping too close to I-20 due to auto noise |
| **Campsites:** | 1.9, 8.0, 9.3, 11.5, 14.8, 17.8, and 19.6 miles |

**CHEAHA TRAILHEAD:** From Exit 191 on I-20 near Anniston, head south on US 431 for 3.6 miles to Cleburne County 131. A sign will indicate "To Talladega Scenic Drive." Turn right on Cleburne County 131 and follow it 0.4 miles to Talladega Scenic Drive, AL 281. Turn left on the Scenic Drive, AL 281, and follow it 11.9 miles to the Cheaha trailhead, which will be on your left.

**CLEBURNE TRAILHEAD:** From Exit 199 on I-20 near Heflin, take AL 9 north for 1.5 miles to US 78. Turn left on US 78 and follow it for

2.6 miles to AL 281, Talladega Scenic Drive. Turn right on the access road for AL 281 and soon come to a four-way intersection. Keep forward here, following signs for FR 500. Drive a short distance, crossing railroad tracks. The Cleburne trailhead is on the right just after the railroad tracks.

This section of trail starts out in Alabama's highest mountains at Cheaha State Park, where it skirts around the actual high point of the state, Cheaha Mountain. The Pinhoti leaves the state park to enter the Talladega National Forest and the Blue Mountain Backcountry Area, soon coming to a fine trail shelter on the shoulder of Blue Mountain. Beyond the shelter, the Pinhoti traces Blue Mountain northward, slowly descending into the Hillabee Creek valley. It is here that the Pinhoti works its way in and out of steep lush hollows nestled in the nooks between forested ridges. Small, clear streams course through these hollows, making their way for Hillabee Creek. The Pinhoti crosses attractive Hillabee Creek itself, then crosses more feeder branches plunging from the hillsides, where waterfalls make melodic interludes in the tranquil forest. Next, the trail makes for Horseblock Mountain on a ridgeline with views before dropping once again into the Hillabee Creek valley. A side trail heads to small Morgan Lake, tucked away in the forest. Beyond Morgan Lake, the Pinhoti continues its hill-and-creek pattern in solitude until it crosses busy US 431. The trail returns to Horseblock Mountain, running along its northwest flank, and passes under I-20. A dip into the Bobo Branch watershed before more ridge running eventually leads to Cleburne and the section's end.

Campsites are numerous in this section. Obviously, water is no problem here. Many of the small creeks have wooded flats suitable for overnighting. Blue Mountain Trail shelter is a viable bad weather option. For a change of pace, Cheaha State Park offers a lodge, cabins, and a campground, all within walking distance of the Pinhoti. There is also a dining room at the lodge and a camp store where picnic and convenience store–type items can be purchased. Campsites with water are at 1.9, 8.0, 9.3, 11.5, 14.8, 17.8, and 19.6 miles. The small town of Heflin, 3 miles from the Cleburne trailhead, avails thru-hikers a chance to resupply at the town's full-service grocery store.

❀   ❀   ❀

Access this segment of the Pinhoti Trail by taking the spur trail ascending from the Cheaha parking area to reach the Pinhoti after the Cave Creek Trail leaves left. Head northbound on the Pinhoti, soon reaching Talladega Scenic Drive. Step down to cross the paved road and re-enter woods. The path now swings around the east side of Cheaha Mountain, coming to a fern-choked stream at 0.4 miles. This is the first of numerous feeder streams of Hillabee Creek that the PT will cross. Climb away and gain views of the mountains to the east. A second stream at 0.8 miles slides down a high rockface. Just past here stands a small rock overhang that could shelter a couple of hikers during a thunderstorm. Roller-coaster steeply up and down before crossing another stream at mile 1.9. Soon, come to the side trail for the Blue Mountain shelter. The side trail leads right 100 yards down to the two-story, wood shingled structure with a picnic table, benches beneath a porch, a main area with open front, and a loft that provides wind protection. The loft is very dark, however. Get your water from the last creek crossed.

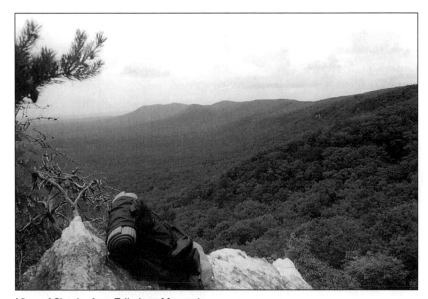

View of Cheaha from Talladega Mountain

The Pinhoti Trail continues forward from the junction, climbing to reach another trail intersection at mile 2.2. At this point you have left the state park and are now in the Blue Mountain Backcountry Area. A side trail ascends left 0.5 miles to Bald Rock, which offers a good view. The state park and its facilities can also be reached via this trail. Make a forest cruise in hickory-oak woods along the slopes of Blue Mountain, gradually descending to reach a gap in the mountain at mile 3.6. Here the trail slips off the ridgeline onto the western slope of the mountain. The Pinhoti continues its gradual descent from the highlands toward hill and creek country, winding into wet weather drainages divided by dry rib ridges. The arrow-straight trunks of tulip trees thrive in the hollows here.

Reach the Oxford-Cheaha Road, FR 589, at mile 4.9. This historic road, built in the 1930s by the Great Depression–era Civilian Conservation Corps, was once the only road to Cheaha State Park. Cross Oxford-Cheaha Road and continue through brushy woods growing from a burn to shortly bisect FR 589A and leave the Blue Mountain Backcountry Area. Drop into a steep drainage, crossing an unnamed branch at mile 6.0. Keep down the creek in the valley, crossing the stream where it pinches in, then walk along the lush valley walls. This creek leads down to another feeder stream that is crossed at mile 6.7. Head up the feeder stream before climbing through low hills, where the trail nears a decades-old jalopy. Pass under a power line just before reaching Hillabee Creek at mile 8.0. This clear stream offers decent smallmouth bass and rock bass fishing. Hillabee Creek can be rock-hopped in times of normal flow.

Traverse Hillabee Creek, then climb a wet-weather drainage, working northeast over a ridgeline. Descend into a lush, intimate drainage, crossing the stream three times before turning up another small stream. Hillabee Creek is just below the confluence of these two branches. The trail here is trying to keep north while working its way through the Hillabee Creek watershed. Continue up the valley, crossing the stream at mile 9.1 and 9.3, as the valley widens to a large flat. Leave the stream, then climb away on an old woods road onto a rib ridge of Horseblock Mountain. Ascend steeply up the piney ridge, aiming east toward Horseblock Mountain. The path levels off, then undulates along the ridge before meeting another woods road at mile 10.3. The Pinhoti Trail makes a conspicuous left turn down this other woods road and generally descends as it rolls northward.

At mile 11.2, a warning sign indicates an old well hole in the ground on trail-left. The trail leaves the roadbed shortly beyond the well hole, dropping right as a footpath down to reach a clear stream and a flat at mile 11.5. Ascend beyond the stream. In times of higher water flow, a cascade can be heard downstream from the crossing. Wind through hills before picking up a small valley that leads to CR 24 at mile 12.1.

Cross the paved county road and immediately come to a creek. A six-foot waterfall cascades just below the trail crossing of this stream. Easy road access has made this pretty spot a party locale—litter may be strewn about. Work your way up this streamshed. Keep an eye open for an unsigned trail junction just ahead. The Pinhoti Trail leads sharply left, switchbacking uphill, while the other trail leads right to the dam at Morgan Lake, a small impoundment. The PT climbs a hill, then ascends a feeder stream of Morgan Lake. Step over the stream twice at mile 12.7, then climb steeply to a ridgeline and level out under broken woods. The Pinhoti crosses old woods roads here and there, but the direction of the trail is clear. Watch for the turkey-track blazes as well as the many up-and-coming longleaf pines in this neck of the woods. The trail then dips into a rocky hollow with a little water. What flow exists drops off many rock ledges. Climb over to the next watershed and the sound of a bona fide waterfall is clearly audible. Cross this stream and come to a side trail leading left to the noisy falls at mile 14.2. The PT continues, and soon reaches another falls, passing by its base where the falls make a 30-foot drop over a rockface. Turn away from this second falls, cross the stream, and wind over to yet another stream, crossing it on a footbridge in a rich flat at mile 14.8. Climb the hollow and reach gravel FR 515 at mile 15.4.

From FR 515, immediately descend into a pretty watershed cloaked in hardwoods, staying far above the creek. Eventually, dip down to cross the creek several times, finally spanning a side stream on a footbridge at mile 16.2. The Pinhoti turns right just beyond the footbridge, up the side stream, and begins climbing toward FR 585, which is reached at mile 16.9. Continue forward, descending the forest road to reach paved US 431 at mile 17.0. Cross the road and turn right, soon heading left back into the woods. Ascend on a single-track path up an intermittent drainage, topping out at mile 17.5. Switchback down to another hollow, then veer left. To your right, at mile 17.8, is a small campsite in a flat alongside a feeder branch of Jackson Creek. A rock bluff lies across the branch.

The Pinhoti Trail keeps north up the feeder branch, briefly following a jeep road. Climb away from the branch and approach a clearing, but turn away to cross FR 518 at mile 18.9. Talladega Scenic Drive is off to your right. Keep northeast on single-track in an oak-hardwood forest. A wooded ravine drops to your left. After crossing a wide jeep track growing up in pines, descend to step over a small stream at mile 19.6. A small campsite lies beside a beech tree just before the stream crossing. Curve back upstream to top a hill and drop to cross another stream at mile 20.0.

Head up and down more hills, all the while angling for I-20. The PT reaches Talladega Scenic Drive at mile 21.3. Turn left on the paved scenic drive, and carefully walk over busy I-20. At mile 21.5, turn right onto a gravel road, then leave left, back onto a single-track path roaming east through the forest. Curve north and cross a gas pipeline clearing at mile 22.1. Stay to the left of the access road. Re-enter woods, paralleling a feeder stream of Bobo Branch. Curve east with the stream, crossing it at mile 22.5. Top a hill, then switchback down to cross a larger feeder branch at mile 22.7. Ascend amid brush to soon cross a second gas pipeline. Work through hills rendered scrubby from fires to reach Talladega Scenic Drive atop Horseblock Mountain at mile 23.5.

Switch over to the west side of Horseblock, leaving the burned woods behind. Descend into a canyon amid mountain laurel, passing a small rock house at mile 23.9. A perennial streamlet flows just beyond the rock house. Circle out of the canyon, turning eastward, passing near a power-line clearing. Bisect a closed forest road at mile 24.8, and descend to pick up a woods road. Turn right on the woods road, still descending, then drop left onto single-track, soon stepping over a small stream above a low-flow fall. Turn upstream and climb, grabbing views to your north and east in a young forest. Pass under two power lines in succession before emerging onto Talladega Scenic Drive at mile 25.7.

Turn left on the scenic drive and cross US 78 below. Keep forward to reach a road junction. Turn right onto FR 500, descending to soon cross the track of Southern Railroad. Take a few steps and reach the Cleburne trailhead at mile 25.9. Ahead, it is 20.1 miles on the Pinhoti Trail to Coleman Lake trailhead. Heflin, which has food and supplies, is about 3 miles east on US 78.

# Pinhoti Trail, Cleburne to Coleman Lake

| | |
|---|---|
| **Length:** | 20.1 miles |
| **Trail Condition:** | Good |
| **Highs:** | Clear streams and lakes, bass fishing, trail shelters, historic church, views |
| **Lows:** | Relatively busy trail segment |
| **Season:** | Year-round, best during spring and fall, though all the water here makes summer more tolerable |
| **Difficulty:** | Moderate |
| **Use:** | Moderate to heavy |
| **Tips:** | Consider bringing fishing rod for stream and lake angling |
| **Campsites:** | 4.6, 7.2, 8.8, 9.7, 12.3, 13.5, 14.4, 15.0, 15.2 16.4, and 16.9 miles |

**CLEBURNE TRAILHEAD:** From Exit 199 on I-20 near Heflin, take AL 9 north for 1.5 miles to US 78. Turn left on US 78 and follow it for 2.6 miles to AL 281, Talladega Scenic Drive. Turn right on the access road for AL 281 and soon come to a four-way intersection. Keep forward here, following signs for FR 500. Drive a short distance, crossing railroad tracks. The Cleburne trailhead is on the right just after the railroad tracks.

**COLEMAN LAKE TRAILHEAD:** From Exit 205 on I-20 take AL 46 to the Shoal Creek Ranger Station on AL 46. From the ranger station, keep forward 0.2 miles on AL 46 to US 78. Turn right on US 78 and follow it for 7.1 miles to Cleburne County 61. Turn left onto Cleburne County 61, at the signs for "National Forest Recreation Areas," as Cleburne County 61 becomes FR 553, for a total of 7.4 miles from US 78. Turn right onto paved FR 500 and follow it 0.3 miles to an intersection. FR 500 turns right again. Follow FR 500 for another 1.1 miles. Coleman Lake trailhead parking will be on your right, just before the Pinhoti Trail crosses FR 500. If you pass the entrance to Coleman Lake Recreation Area, you have gone too far.

This trail segment was my introduction to the Pinhoti Trail many years ago. Here, the Pinhoti leaves the Cleburne trailhead and works along a ridgeline over Brymer Mountain, toward the streams and lakes of the Shoal Creek watershed. Reach the Lower Shoal trail shelter in an attractive wooded flat where two creeks converge. The path temporarily leaves the water, only to follow the larger stream near spacious meadow-like wildlife clearings and through rich beech bottoms. Meet quiet Highrock Lake before arriving at the campground of Pine Glen Recreation Area. From here, the Pinhoti heads upstream along Shoal Creek, which offers first-rate bass fishing among its pools and rapids. The fishing is also good at Sweetwater Lake, where Shoal Creek is dammed. The path continues up Shoal Creek and makes Laurel trail shelter. Beyond this shelter, the Pinhoti winds over low hills to reach historic Shoal Creek Church, built from hand-hewn logs in the 1800s. North of the church, the Pinhoti circles Coleman Lake, the final damming of Shoal Creek. Finally, the path climbs through pine-wiregrass woods to reach the Coleman Lake trailhead.

Campsite options range from backcountry sites to trail shelters to a developed campground. Campsites with water are located at 4.6, 8.8, 9.7, 13.5, 14.4, 15.0, 15.2, and 16.9 miles. Trail shelters with water are located at 7.2 and 16.4 miles. Pine Glen Campground is located at 12.3 miles.

❁    ❁    ❁

Leave north from the Cleburne trailhead and enter a small flat with pine and tulip trees. Span a small stream on a footlog. Upstream is a potential campsite for late night trailhead arrivals. Climb a hill away from the flat and cross FR 500. Begin a generally northward course, passing near a timbered hillside. Ascend a piney hill, gaining views to the west, beyond the Choccolocco Creek watershed. Begin a pattern of winding in hollows and around rib ridges on the west side of the unnamed north-south ridgeline, essentially a northward extension of Horseblock Mountain.

At 0.8 miles, cross an intermittent streambed in a hollow. Pines become more prevalent as the trail extends onto a south-facing rib ridge. A burned over area offers southward views all the way to Cheaha Mountain. Maples thrive on the moister north facing sides of the rib ridges, while oaks grow throughout the mountainside. Pass over intermittent streambeds at miles 1.3 and 1.7. Ascend to a knob of longleaf pines and reach a southwesterly view from a short side trail leading left. Keep north along a steep side slope to reach another streambed at mile 2.6. More westward views await on the next piney rib ridge. Dip down to one more hollow before reaching gravel FR 523 at mile 3.3. This forest road runs along the east-west ridgeline of Brymer Mountain.

Descend north from FR 523, entering the Choccolocco Wildlife Management Area. Not long afterwards, turn eastward, again winding in and out of hollows, and approach a view in a stand of shortleaf pines. At mile 4.6, after circling a shallow valley, the Pinhoti Trail turns west and passes a perennial stream (the headwaters of Joseph Creek), below to the left. Potential campsites can be found if you follow the stream down to larger flats below. Circle around a knob to emerge onto FR 531 at mile 6.1.

Cross the forest road and enter the Shoal Creek watershed. The Pinhoti begins working toward Lower Shoal shelter. Pass an area of many fallen trees, the aftermath of fire. At mile 6.8, the trail makes a U-turn to the left and descends along an unnamed stream to reach the Lower Shoal trail shelter at mile 7.2. Mountain laurel and hardwoods landscape the flat created where two creeks merge. The three-sided shelter has an overhanging roof and sleeps six. A picnic table and fire ring are nearby.

The PT passes behind the shelter, then crosses the adjacent stream, which can be rock-hopped most times of the year. Briefly head up the valley of the larger converging streams, then leave left up a steep hollow to reach the ridgeline and pick up a woods road. Here, the PT turns right, briefly tracing the road to leave left again as a single-track footpath. Follow the ridgeline north in broken-canopied woods between streamsheds. At mile 7.9, the PT crosses an old woods road in an obvious gap. The trail then works downhill on a precipitous bluff to reach an unnamed creek at mile 8.8. The beech-oak flat has a grassy understory and makes for a good campsite.

The PT continues forward, crossing the unnamed creek, which can be easily dry-footed, to turn upstream and ascend a hill. Here, the path bisects an old woods road and returns northbound, cruising on the hillside above a huge flat on the left. At mile 9.0, step over a tiny branch and keep alongside the hill. Eventually drop down to the Shoal Creek feeder branch and appreciate the water clarity. Don't be surprised if you see beaver dams in the area. The Pinhoti curves eastward into the valley of another feeder stream. Rock-hop this branch at mile 9.7, though it could be a wet ford in times of higher flow, and find another large flat with campsites. Curve out of the hollow, shortly spanning a streamlet via a wooden bridge. The Pinhoti ascends away from this attractive area to split a gap, then dip to cross a small creek, reaching FR 531 at mile 10.1.

The PT extends beyond the forest road, and circles around a small creek, then reaches the wetlands forming the upper end of Highrock Lake. Built by the Soil Conservation Service in the 1950s and now known as the Natural Resources Conservation Service, the purpose of these watershed lakes was to provide rural water services and guard against drought.

Turn away from the lake to reach a jeep track, which leads left, back to the lake. The PT turns right on the jeep track and follows it a short distance, then veers left onto a high bluff overlooking the upper end of the slender impoundment. Leave Highrock Lake on the PT to near FR 531-E at mile 10.9. Stay on the bluff as Shoal Creek curves away, then back, then away again, while the Pinhoti continues eastward.

At mile 11.6, a large meadow-like wildlife clearing becomes visible to your left, as the Pinhoti drops near creek elevation. Pass through an extremely attractive beech grove with a grassy understory. Step over a small feeder stream at mile 12.0, just before reaching Shoal Creek and the closed forest road used to maintain the wildlife clearings. Turn away from Shoal Creek and climb a hill, gaining glimpses of Pine Glen campground, which offers drinking water. The Pinhoti reaches FR 500 at mile 12.3. Turn left on FR 500, passing the campground, and cross Shoal Creek on a road bridge.

Just after the bridge, the PT turns right, heading upstream along Shoal Creek. Enjoy the bottomland hardwood-forest mixed with tall pines, beard cane and mountain laurel. The walking is easy as you pass a wildlife clearing on your left at mile 12.8. Campsites are abundant throughout this section, as one side or the other of Shoal Creek has wide flats.

The Pinhoti Trail climbs a hillside while cutting across a wide bend in Shoal Creek. Pass through a shady gap at mile 14.1, soon reaching the flats of Shoal Creek again. At mile 14.4, span a feeder branch on a plank bridge. Leave the streamside flat once again, reaching a grassy field overlooking Sweetwater Lake at mile 14.7. Sweetwater Lake is the largest

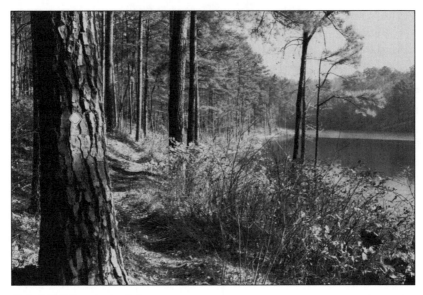

Pinhoti Trail, Sweetwater Lake

impoundment in the northern half of the Talladega National Forest. The dam is off to your right. Keep forward, crossing the field and re-enter forest on the west shore of the lake. At mile 15.0, cut through a peninsula jutting into the lake. A nice campsite is nearby. Reach the auto access and boat ramp for the lake at mile 15.1. Keep along the western shore, circling around a small arm of the lake. The Pinhoti crosses a small branch feeding the lake and enters a small, sloped campsite. Keep along the west bank of Sweetwater Lake, turning away from the lake at mile 15.6. Bisect a horse trail three times before reaching a high point and descending into a hollow to cross a large feeder branch of Shoal Creek. This crossing could be wet in spring. Just across the stream, at mile 16.4, stands the Laurel Trail Shelter. The three-sided, shed-roofed affair sleeps six campers. It overlooks a small flat and has a picnic table and fire ring.

The Pinhoti veers left away from the shelter, then heads north up a low hill. For the next few miles the terrain is gentler, with rolling hills and shallow valleys. Dip to reach two small streams just above their confluence in a potential camping flat at mile 16.9. Turn up the second creek in a shallow valley, spanning a small gullied streamlet on a wooden bridge. Meander through gently rolling terrain, passing a wildlife clearing on your right, then walk under a power line, before reaching paved FR 553 at mile 17.8.

The single-track PT continues forward, passing near historic Shoal Creek Church at mile 18.2. Built of hand-hewn logs between 1885 and 1890, this church was preceded by another one built in 1823. A cemetery and sheltered picnic tables add to the site. The Pinhoti soon crosses FR 553-D, then keeps northwest for Coleman Lake, soon crossing a bridle path. The PT turns away from FR 553-D at a loblolly pine–progeny test site. Coleman Lake shortly comes into view. Turn left and circle around a hollow, spanning a lake feeder branch on a plank bridge at mile 18.9. A recreation trail circling Coleman Lake lies to your right. Roughly follow the west bank of Coleman Lake and drop down to span a second lake feeder branch on a metal bridge at mile 19.8. A nice camping flat lies here. The Pinhoti leaves the flat for widely separated pines with a high grass understory.

Reach a trail junction at mile 20.1. A short side trail leads left to the Coleman Lake trailhead parking. The Pinhoti Trail keeps forward to shortly reach FR 500. This segment of the Pinhoti Trail ends here.

# Pinhoti Trail, Coleman Lake to East Dugger Mountain

| | |
|---|---|
| **Length:** | 15.3 miles |
| **Trail Condition:** | Mostly good |
| **Highs:** | Dugger Mountain Wilderness, views aplenty, solitude, Pinky Burns cabin |
| **Lows:** | Possible ford of creek, limited water last half of hike |
| **Season:** | Spring, fall, and winter |
| **Difficulty:** | Fairly difficult |
| **Use:** | Light to moderate |
| **Tips:** | Plan for slow travel atop Dugger Mountain |
| **Campsites:** | 2.7, 2.9, 3.7, 6.3, 9.8, and 14.8 miles |

**COLEMAN LAKE TRAILHEAD:** From Exit 205 on I-20, take AL 46 to the Shoal Creek Ranger Station on AL 46. From the ranger station, keep forward 0.2 miles on AL 46 to US 78. Turn right on US 78 east and follow it for 7.1 miles to Cleburne County 61. Turn left onto Cleburne County 61, at the sign for "National Forest Recreation Areas," as Cleburne County 61 becomes FR 553, for a total of 7.4 miles from US 78. Turn right onto paved FR 500 and follow it 0.3 miles to an intersection. FR 500 turns right again. Follow FR 500 for 1.1 more miles. Coleman Lake trailhead parking will be on your right, just before the Pinhoti Trail crosses FR 500. If you pass the entrance to Coleman Lake Recreation Area you have gone too far.

**EAST DUGGER MOUNTAIN TRAILHEAD:**
From the junction of US 278 and AL 9 in Piedmont, drive south on AL 9 for 0.8 miles to Ladiga Street, which is just before AL 21. Turn left on Ladiga Street, passing through old downtown Piedmont, keeping forward for 3.3 miles to Hebble Highway. Turn right on Hebble Highway, crossing the Chief Ladiga Rail Trail and follow Hebble Highway for 0.3 miles to Dugger Mountain Road. Turn left on Dugger Mountain Road, which becomes FR 500 after 1.4 miles. The forest road becomes gravel within 1.2 miles. FR 500 crosses the Pinhoti Trail 3.4 miles from Hebble Highway. Small signs on both sides of the road mark the trail. The trailhead is on the right just after passing the Pinhoti Trail.

This trail segment features the federally designated Dugger Mountain Wilderness. The path begins innocently enough in low pine hills before dropping into the attractive upper Choccolocco Creek watershed. The walking remains easy as the PT passes Choccolocco Lake. Then things change. Enter the Dugger Mountain Wilderness and ascend Red Mountain. Great views await of Dugger Mountain and the Jones Branch watershed. Keep climbing to reach the crest of Dugger Mountain, Alabama's second highest peak. Plenty of views open up among the trees and rocks. Descend off the mountain to reach a quiet stream, now in the Terrapin Creek watershed, and reach FR 500.

Dugger Mountain was named for Thomas Dugger, a Civil War veteran who moved here from Tennessee, and homesteaded at the foot of the mountain. The mountain was later purchased by the Forest Service, which managed Dugger Mountain as a wilderness study area. Finally, in late 1999, Congress declared the 9,200-acre area a federally designated wilderness.

Campsites are evenly spread throughout this trail segment and offer a variety of environments, from streamside and lakeside camps to high and dry wilderness sites. The ups and downs are much more frequent and challenging along the last half of the section. Campsites with water are located at 2.7, 2.9, 3.7, 6.3, 9.8, and 14.8 miles.

❈    ❈    ❈

Reach the Pinhoti Trail by heading south on a short access trail from the Coleman Lake parking area. Turn left, north, on the Pinhoti and soon cross FR 500. Enter a woodland of widely separated pines and an understory of wiregrass and scrub oak. The open forest lays bare the topography of the land. The PT heads for a bank of young pines then turns away, curving around the side of Abernathy Mountain, which looks more like a mountain from the northern side. White quartz rock lies scattered on the ground below. These open pines are favorable habitat for the red cockaded woodpecker.

Turn north to split a gap and bridle path at mile 1.3. The PT works around a hillside to reach gravel FR 540 at mile 1.7. Cross the road and descend into the Choccolocco Creek watershed on a single-track path in a hardwood forest. The water-carved valley soon becomes steeper and deeper.

The PT descends to join the main stream as it slices through a steep, rock-walled canyon. Step over the stream at miles 2.5 and 2.7. A campsite lies just after this second crossing. Soon step over a side branch and cross the main stream again at mile 2.9. You are now on the right streambank at another small campsite near the mountain laurel–lined creek. The PT passes a small rock house, then ascends over a scrubby bluff into young hardwood forest. Shortly, cross another bridle path and pick up an old roadbed that makes for easy walking.

At mile 3.2, step over an unnamed creek coming in from your right. At mile 3.7, the Pinhoti reaches a large flat. Look around for old washtubs and other evidence of a former homesite. The path crosses the main stream just beyond here, which will wet boots in times of normal to high flow. In the flats around the stream look for wallowings and dug up ground—boar sign. The PT resumes the old roadbed and curves to the south. Look for beaver dams along the creek. At mile 4.2, the Pinhoti abruptly leaves the roadbed left, and heads sharply up a narrow valley on a single-track path. Switchback onto a precipitous hillside, roughly paralleling the stream far below. The PT then circles a hickory-laden knob with a small streamshed to the left, and passes through a gap at mile 4.9.

Work toward Choccolocco Watershed Lake. Its backwaters become visible before reaching a pine bluff overlooking the lake. The Pinhoti Trail then emerges onto a field at mile 5.9 and crosses the lake dam, which offers good lake views, then makes a sharp right, re-entering woods, and parallels the lake far above the shoreline. A lakeside camp lies below at mile 6.3, but you must scramble down a steep slope to access it.

At mile 6.5, the PT leaves the lake and heads up along small streamlet. Get water here, as there is no reliable source for several miles. At mile 7.3, reach CR 55, Rabbittown Road. To your left is the old Pinky Burns Cabin, which is owned by the Forest Service and is slated for rehab and trailhead parking. Ol' Pinky never owned the cabin, but obtained it in a perpetuity lease from the Savage family, who built the original part of the cabin as a schoolhouse for their many children. Pinky's father later moved into the cabin, adding on to what you see today. The last Burns left the area, then the Forest Service acquired the property.

The Pinhoti Trail crosses Rabbittown Road and enters the Dugger Mountain Wilderness. The trail is irregularly blazed in the wilderness, so watch carefully for the path. Make a short descent into a shallow valley, then begin climbing. Head up Red Mountain, soon making a rock bluff dominated by shortleaf pine and chestnut oaks. At mile 8.3, split a gap in the ridge.

Head north, on the west side of the ridgeline, winding in and out of numerous intermittent streamsheds. The crest and rugged bluffs of Dugger Mountain are visible to the northwest across the Jones Branch valley. The area exudes a grand and wild aura. At mile 9.8, reach the gap dividing Red Mountain from Dugger Mountain. An old, closed forest road cuts through the gap, coming up from Jones Branch to your left and heading over to the valley to your right. This roadbed is slated to be part of a Dugger Mountain trail system in the future. For now, you can take the old forest road right about 200 yards to reach a perennial stream and level area suitable for camping. Campsites and water can also be found left, down Jones Branch, although you must travel farther down the valley to reach water.

The Pinhoti Trail continues up Dugger Mountain, climbing out of the gap. At mile 10.2, swing around an obvious outcrop to your left and keep climbing to step over a tiny spring branch at mile 10.5. Water can be accessed just below the trail. Keep climbing to reach a gap between Dugger Mountain and a rib ridge to the right at mile 10.9. A dry campsite is in the gap. Veer left in maples to reach a gap in the main crest of Dugger Mountain at mile 11.1. The Pinhoti ascends northeast on a rocky and sometimes faint trailbed. Enjoy occasional views of the mountains and valleys to your west from atop Dugger. Drift over to the north side of the mountain and look down on the town of Piedmont.

Regain the crest of the ridge at mile 12.0. Occasionally, piled rocks—rock cairns—mark the trail. Keep in a northeasterly direction, reaching a gap in the ridge at mile 12.4. Head back over to the north side of the ridge. Shortly reach another gap and circle around the south side of Dugger Mountain's high point of 2,140 feet. Good views abound to the south and east amid the pines.

At mile 13.2, pass between two rocky knobs, switching to the north side of Dugger Mountain yet again. Begin to seriously drop off the mountain in a dense stand of pines at mile 14.1. Hardwoods become more prevalent upon entering the stream valley below. At mile 14.8, step over a perennial stream. Flats suitable for camping are in the area. Step over the stream again at mile 15.0 and 15.1. Cross a feeder branch of the main stream just before leaving the Dugger Mountain Wilderness, reaching FR 500 and the end of this trail segment at mile 15.3.

# Pinhoti Trail, East Dugger Mountain to High Point

| | |
|---|---|
| **Length:** | 15.3 miles |
| **Trail Condition:** | Good |
| **Highs:** | Views, solitude, Chief Ladiga Rail Trail, waterfall |
| **Lows:** | Rocky trail, numerous ups and downs |
| **Season:** | Spring, fall, and winter |
| **Difficulty:** | Fairly difficult |
| **Use:** | Light to moderate |
| **Tips:** | Be mentally prepared for many ups and downs |
| **Campsites:** | 2.9, 5.0, and 13.6 miles |

**EAST DUGGER MOUNTAIN TRAILHEAD:** From the junction of US 278 and AL 9 in Piedmont, drive south on AL 9 for 0.8 miles to Ladiga Street, which is just before AL 21. Turn left on Ladiga Street, passing through old downtown Piedmont, keeping forward for 3.3 miles to Hebble Highway. Turn right on Hebble Highway, crossing the Chief Ladiga Rail Trail and follow Hebble Highway for 0.3 miles to Dugger Mountain Road. Turn left on Dugger Mountain Road, which becomes FR 500 after 1.4 miles. The forest road becomes gravel 1.2 miles farther on. Forest Road 500 crosses the Pinhoti Trail 3.4 miles from Hebble Highway. Small signs on both sides of the road mark the trail. The trailhead is on the right just after passing the Pinhoti Trail.

**HIGH POINT TRAILHEAD:** From the junction of US 278 and AL 9 in Piedmont, drive east on US 278 for 9 miles. The trailhead is on the right. A small sign marks the Pinhoti Trail on US 278.

This trail segment encompasses some of the newer sections of the Pinhoti, as it makes its way north to the end of the national forest and currently the most northerly-located public parking access. Most of the hiking is on ridgetops, broken by descents to valleys, followed by another climb to a ridgeline. Leave a quiet valley at the eastern foot of Dugger Mountain and climb an unnamed mountain, only to drop back to Terrapin Watershed Lake. From here, make a winding ascent up the steep slopes of Oakey Mountain. Dip to a quiet valley, ideal for camping, then head northeast, enjoying views along a ridgeline before dropping down to the deep Terrapin Creek valley, passing a waterfall along the way. Here, the Pinhoti joins the Chief Ladiga Rail Trail, crossing Terrapin Creek on an old railroad trestle. Resume climbing up the south-facing, sun-scorched Wilson Ridge, only to drop to Maxwell Gap. Make another south-facing ascent up the side of Augusta Mine Ridge, cresting out at nearly 1,900 feet. The northeast end of the ridge becomes a little confusing before the PT drops to Lanie Gap, circles around the east side of Wolf Ridge, and begins an extended descent along the slopes of Rock Quarry Mountain to make Lanie Hollow. Squeeze through the lower portion of Lanie Hollow as it narrows into a tight valley before opening near High Point and the end of the segment on US 278.

The ridges on this section are generally rocky, making the going slow. The ups and downs can wear down a heavily loaded backpacker. Water is virtually nonexistent up high—you must plan your watering holes and camping locales more carefully than the previous trail segments. However, this more challenging trek offers increased solitude. Campsites with water are located at 2.9, 5.0, and 13.6 miles.

❀　　❀　　❀

Start this trail segment by leaving FR 500 and heading northeast up an intermittent drainage. Step over the streambed and continue uphill through burned woods. Jump over a rib ridge on a single-track path, crossing a firebreak heading straight up and down the ridge at 0.5 miles. Angle up the rocky ridgeline. South Fork Terrapin Creek valley is down to your right. Reach the rocky ridgecrest at 0.8 miles. Head northeast along a rock-lined path. The trail is fairly level, but the rocky treadway makes the going slow on the faint, rock-strewn path. At mile 1.1, the Pinhoti picks up a wide roadbed, but shortly leaves left, back on single-track, descending toward Terrapin Watershed Lake, which becomes visible by mile 1.8. Steep Oakey Mountain forms the lake's backdrop. Descend by switchbacks on a precipitous pine-studded slope and open onto a field at mile 2.1. Turn right and cross the dam of Terrapin Watershed Lake.

Re-enter woods at mile 2.3, climbing into a maze of downed trees resembling a war zone. This is a result of Hurricane Opal, which passed through here in 1995. The Pinhoti circles down to a feeder branch of

South Fork Terrapin Creek at mile 2.9. A small, sloped campsite lies near the creek. Turn east up the valley, crossing an intermittent streambed at mile 3.1. Pick up the ridgeline, angling upward on the steep northwest slope of Oakey Mountain. Make every step count on the slender foot-bed. Little Tank Ridge and Big Tank Ridge are visible across the Terrapin Creek Valley. Oakey Mountain becomes rockier as the Pinhoti nears the crest, which is reached at mile 4.5. Immediately descend to the increasingly piney south slope, which offers scattered views to the southeast. Pass a national-forest boundary marker before reaching an isolated and high valley flat at mile 5.0. This flat offers good camping and solitude. The path turns left here, briefly picking up a roadbed. Water is available from a small creek below the roadbed.

The PT leaves the roadbed and begins circling around a high knob, crossing an ATV trail. Good views lie ahead in the sparse pines and oaks growing amid scattered rock gardens. At mile 5.7, cross another ATV trail, keeping north to cross over a rocky rib ridge. Enter a dense stand of shortleaf pines, then begin descending toward Terrapin Creek down an unnamed small stream valley. This is your last chance for good mountain water for 7 miles, so fill up here. At mile 6.5, pass a 10-foot waterfall dropping over a sheer rock bluff to your right.

The Pinhoti turns away from the streambed and drifts down low hills, crossing a dirt road just before reaching the Chief Ladiga Rail Trail at mile 7.4. Turn right on the dirt-and-gravel rail right-of-way. Its wide, straight, and level character contrasts greatly with the single-track, winding, and undulating Pinhoti you have been tracing. Shortly, span big Terrapin Creek on a restored railroad trestle. At mile 8.0, the Pinhoti leaves left from the rail trail and re-enters woods, soon crossing quiet CR 94. Ascend gently away from the road, crossing a firebreak from a late 2001 blaze. Soon, leave the burned area as the ascent sharpens onto a piney ridge, where views open to the south of Oakey Mountain. At mile 8.7, the Pinhoti curves north, heading for a gap in Wilson Ridge. Pass an intermittent spring before reaching the gap at mile 9.1. Keep north, passing over a rocky rib ridge, then angle downhill, reaching Maxwell Gap at mile 9.6.

The Pinhoti crosses CR 70 at Maxwell Gap and begins angling up a dry, piney slope toward the southwest end of Augusta Mine Ridge. At mile 9.9, the PT curves sharply right and keeps climbing, soon offering sporadic views to the east. At mile 10.4, pass a rock outcrop to your left, with views open to the east. Shortly, drop to a gap in the ridgeline and resume climbing, reaching a high point at mile 10.8. Undulate along the ridgeline, staying with the blue blazes, and pass a plaque commemorating a trail easement grant at mile 11.2. Beyond here, two rock-lined paths diverge—the Pinhoti stays with the upper path keeping along the ridgeline.

More southeastward views await on the ridgeline. At mile 11.6, make a sharp turn to the left, leaving Augusta Mine Ridge and angling toward Lanie Gap. An ATV trail keeps forward. Hardwoods predominate on the moister, north-facing mountainside. Reach Lanie Gap and a dry campsite at mile 11.9. Veer right from the gap, staying on a single-track footpath, avoiding the jeep roads diverging from the gap. Head north along the east flank of Wolf Ridge, slipping across a flat and to the west side of the ridgeline at mile 12.4. The Pinhoti then works around a small knob to the east.

At mile 12.7, make a sharp switchback to the right and head east down a gently sloping ridgeline. Reach an intermittent streambed on the slopes of Rock Quarry Mountain at mile 13.2. Briefly pick up a roadbed, leaving left again as a single-track path. Circle around a rib ridge to reach a perennial stream at mile 13.6. The flat below has camping potential. Keep in a northeasterly direction, entering a thicker forest amid old mining pits at mile 14.1. These pits may have been for iron ore, graphite gravel, or gold mining, all of which took place in the area in times past. Graphite was used during World War II to make crucibles, large heat resistant containers from which molten metals are poured into casts to make tanks and other machines of war.

Descend to near a dirt road on your right, passing through more manipulated and dug land. The Pinhoti crosses Lanie Hollow Branch, where the valley has constricted at mile 14.6. Keep north, looking down on the stream for an old concrete dam. The creek falls away as the Pinhoti keeps on the west flank of High Point. The hollow opens and the Pinhoti continues through young woods on a grassy footbed to reach the parking area at US 278 at mile 15.3. The Pinhoti Trail is currently being extended to the Georgia state line and beyond to intersect the Benton MacKaye Trail, which will ultimately make a journey from Alabama to Maine viable.

## Pinhoti Trail Log

### PORTERS GAP TO CHEAHA STATE PARK

| | | |
|---|---|---|
| **0.0** | **102.9** | Beginning of Pinhoti Trail at near Porters Gap |
| **1.4** | **101.5** | Chandler Gap |
| **3.2** | **99.7** | Descend to CR 394. Turn left onto paved road |
| **3.4** | **99.5** | Cross railroad tracks, then Talladega Creek on road bridge |
| **3.6** | **99.3** | Bridge Clear Creek on footbridge followed by long boardwalk |
| **3.7** | **99.2** | Reach gravel FR 249, keep in hills |
| **4.8** | **98.1** | Cross FR 600-2. Keep forward on foot trail |
| **5.1** | **97.8** | Reach perennial stream, only water for over 7 miles |
| **6.0** | **96.9** | Cross FR 600-2. Keep northeast on very rocky trail |
| **8.7** | **94.2** | Clairmont Gap. Ascend to ridgecrest and views of Talladega Creek. Travel north slope of mountain |
| **11.1** | **91.8** | Cross FR 600-2. Swing around Burgess Point |
| **11.9** | **91.0** | Cross FR 600-2. Keep north along Talladega Mountain |
| **13.2** | **89.7** | Cross FR 6230. Descend to stream |
| **15.2** | **87.7** | Trail junction. Skyway Loop Trail leads left to Lake Chinnabee |
| **15.3** | **87.6** | Adams Gap. Trail crosses Talladega Scenic Drive and enters Cheaha Wilderness |
| **16.5** | **86.4** | Step over stream on north slope of Talladega Mountain |
| **18.8** | **84.1** | Signed right turn begins steep climb of Talladega Mountain |
| **19.7** | **83.2** | Trail reaches crest of Talladega Mountain after steep climb, attaining 2,000 feet. Continue on Alabama's highest ridgecrest |
| **21.3** | **81.6** | Intersect Chinnabee Silent Trail and Odum Trail in popular camping area near spring |
| **22.8** | **80.1** | Trail junction. Cave Creek Trail leads right. Pinhoti veers left into boulder field |
| **24.2** | **78.7** | Side trail leads left to McDill Overlook |
| **25.2** | **77.7** | Reach top of Hernandez Peak at 2,344 feet, highest point on entire Pinhoti Trail |
| **26.3** | **76.6** | Reach trail junction. Side trail leads right short distance to Cheaha trailhead parking. |

### CHEAHA STATE PARK TO CLEBURNE

| | | |
|---|---|---|
| **26.7** | **76.2** | First of two streams flowing off side of Cheaha |
| **28.2** | **74.7** | Cross water source for Blue Mountain trail shelter |
| **28.3** | **74.6** | Side trail leads right to Blue Mountain trail shelter |
| **28.5** | **74.4** | Side trail leads left to Bald Rock and Cheaha State Park facilities |
| **29.9** | **73.0** | Reach gap in Blue Mountain. Descend to hill and creek country |
| **31.2** | **71.7** | Cross historic Oxford-Cheaha Road |

## Pinhoti Trail Log *(continued)*

| | | |
|---|---|---|
| **34.3** | **68.6** | Cross Hillabee Creek, ascend away from stream |
| **35.6** | **67.3** | Leave streambed and ascend on woods road |
| **36.9** | **66.0** | Meet second woods road. Abruptly turn left |
| **37.5** | **65.4** | Pass old well hole on left. Warning sign |
| **37.8** | **65.1** | Descend to reach clear stream and flat |
| **38.4** | **64.5** | Cross paved CR 24. Descend to waterfall |
| **39.0** | **63.9** | Step over stream feeding Morgan Lake |
| **40.5** | **62.4** | Side trail leads left to waterfall. Second waterfall just ahead |
| **41.1** | **61.8** | Span small stream on footbridge with handrails |
| **41.7** | **61.2** | Cross gravel FR 515 |
| **42.5** | **60.4** | Turn right up hollow after crossing wood footbridge |
| **43.2** | **59.7** | Reach FR 585. Keep forward and descend on gravel road |
| **43.3** | **59.6** | Cross US 431. Climb drainage |
| **44.1** | **58.8** | Small campsite in flat along creek |
| **45.2** | **57.7** | Cross FR 518 |
| **45.9** | **57.0** | Step over small stream, small campsite nearby |
| **46.3** | **56.6** | Step over small stream |
| **47.6** | **55.3** | Reach Talladega Scenic Drive. Use drive to span I-20 |
| **47.9** | **55.0** | Turn right onto gravel road, shortly leave left on single-track trail |
| **48.5** | **54.4** | Cross gas pipeline clearing |
| **48.9** | **54.0** | Step over feeder stream of Bob Branch, soon cross second feeder branch |
| **49.9** | **53.0** | Cross Talladega Scenic Drive |
| **50.2** | **52.7** | Descend into canyon and pass small rock house |
| **51.1** | **51.8** | Cross closed forest road, descend to stream with small waterfall |
| **52.0** | **50.9** | Reach Talladega Scenic Drive. Turn left on scenic drive and span US 78 |
| **52.2** | **50.7** | Reach Cleburne trailhead after following FR 500 for a short distance and crossing Southern Railroad tracks |

## CLEBURNE TO COLEMAN LAKE

| | | |
|---|---|---|
| **53.0** | **49.9** | Step over intermittent streambed while heading along north-south ridge, views ahead |
| **53.3** | **49.6** | Cross intermittent streambed, wind along ridge |
| **55.5** | **47.4** | Cross FR 523 on Brymer Mountain |
| **56.8** | **46.1** | Headwaters of Joseph Creek, potential campsites down hollow |
| **58.3** | **44.6** | Cross FR 531 |
| **59.0** | **43.9** | PT makes U-turn, descends into Shoal Creek watershed |
| **59.4** | **43.5** | Reach Lower Shoal trail shelter |
| **60.1** | **42.8** | Bisect old woods road in obvious gap |

## Pinhoti Trail Log *(continued)*

| | | |
|---|---|---|
| **61.0** | **41.9** | Cross unnamed creek, campsite |
| **61.9** | **41.0** | Rock-hop feeder branch, flat with campsites |
| **62.3** | **40.6** | Cross FR 531, soon near Highrock Lake |
| **63.1** | **39.8** | Near FR 531-E |
| **63.8** | **39.1** | Meadow-like wildlife clearing becomes visible across stream |
| **64.2** | **38.7** | Step over small feeder stream at Shoal Creek |
| **64.5** | **38.4** | Reach FR 500. Pine Glen campground to your left. Cross forest road bridge over Shoal Creek and turn upstream |
| **65.0** | **37.9** | Pass wildlife clearing on your left, keep upstream along Shoal Creek |
| **66.3** | **36.6** | Bisect gap as Shoal Creek makes wide bend away from PT |
| **66.6** | **36.3** | Span feeder stream on plank bridge in streamside flat |
| **66.9** | **36.0** | Reach grassy field overlooking Sweetwater Lake |
| **67.2** | **35.7** | Cut across lake peninsula, campsite |
| **67.3** | **35.6** | Reach auto access road and boat ramp for Sweetwater Lake, small, sloped campsite ahead near lake feeder branch |
| **67.8** | **35.1** | Turn away from Sweetwater Lake |
| **68.6** | **34.3** | Reach Laurel trail shelter after crossing feeder branch of Shoal Creek |
| **69.1** | **33.8** | Camping flat at confluence of two small streams |
| **70.0** | **32.9** | Cross paved FR 553 |
| **70.4** | **32.5** | Pass historic Shoal Creek Church, hewn log church, cemetery, sheltered picnic tables |
| **71.1** | **31.8** | Span feeder branch of Coleman Lake on plank footbridge |
| **72.0** | **30.9** | Span second lake feeder branch, camping flat |
| **72.3** | **30.6** | Trail junction. Access trail leaves left to Coleman Lake trailhead. Pinhoti keeps forward to shortly cross FR 500. East Dugger Mountain trailhead 15.3 miles ahead |

## COLEMAN LAKE TO EAST DUGGER MOUNTAIN

| | | |
|---|---|---|
| **73.6** | **29.3** | Split gap after climbing through low hills |
| **74.0** | **28.9** | Cross FR 540, descend into Choccolocco Creek watershed |
| **74.8** | **28.1** | Step over stream for first of three times, campsites in area |
| **76.0** | **26.9** | Cross unnamed stream you have been following, possible ford. Large flat in area that was once homesite |
| **76.5** | **26.4** | PT leaves sharply left off old roadbed, climbs away from stream |
| **78.2** | **24.7** | Enter field adjacent to Choccolocco Watershed Lake |
| **78.6** | **24.3** | Difficult-to-access lakeside camp |
| **78.8** | **24.1** | Leave lake up streambed, small stream |

## Pinhoti Trail Log *(continued)*

| | | |
|---|---|---|
| **79.6** | **23.3** | Cross CR 55, Rabbittown Road, historic Pinky Burns Cabin to left, enter Dugger Mountain Wilderness, heading up Red Mountain |
| **80.6** | **22.3** | Split gap in the ridge |
| **82.1** | **20.8** | Gap between Red Mountain and Dugger Mountain. Old jeep road splits gap. Jones Branch valley to left, water and campsite to right 200 yards |
| **82.8** | **20.1** | Tiny spring branch just below trail |
| **83.1** | **19.8** | Reach gap between Dugger Mountain and rib ridge to right |
| **83.3** | **19.6** | Reach main crest of Dugger Mountain, ascend northeast on rocky trailbed |
| **84.7** | **18.2** | Swing over to north side of ridge in gap, near high point of mountain |
| **85.5** | **17.4** | Pass between two rocky knobs |
| **86.4** | **16.5** | Begin to seriously drop off mountain in dense pine stand |
| **87.1** | **15.8** | Step over perennial stream, first of three times, campsites in area |
| **87.6** | **15.3** | Cross FR 500, trailside parking to the right. PT keeps forward up intermittent drainage |

### EAST DUGGER MOUNTAIN TO HIGH POINT

| | | |
|---|---|---|
| **88.4** | **14.5** | Reach crest of unnamed ridge |
| **89.7** | **13.2** | Cross field and dam of Terrapin Watershed Lake |
| **90.5** | **12.4** | Reach feeder branch of South Fork Terrapin Creek, small, sloped campsite |
| **92.1** | **10.8** | Reach crest of Oakey Mountain, descend onto piney slope |
| **92.6** | **10.3** | Small stream and campsite in high, isolated flat. PT swings around knob |
| **94.1** | **8.8** | Pass 10-foot low-flow waterfall while descending toward Terrapin Creek. Last water for 7 miles |
| **95.0** | **7.9** | PT turns right, running in conjunction with Chief Ladiga Rail Trail |
| **95.6** | **7.3** | Leave rail trail after spanning Terrapin Creek on trestle, soon cross CR 94, then ascend Wilson Ridge |
| **96.7** | **6.2** | Split gap in Wilson Ridge, descend |
| **97.2** | **5.7** | Cross CR 70 at Maxwell Gap, ascend Augusta Mine Ridge |
| **98.4** | **4.5** | Reach high point on ridge, views in area |
| **98.8** | **4.1** | Pass plaque commemorating trail easement |
| **99.2** | **3.7** | Angle down toward Lanie Gap after gaining more ridgetop vistas |
| **99.5** | **3.4** | Lanie Gap, dry campsite. PT stays as footpath avoiding jeep tracks |

## Pinhoti Trail Log *(continued)*

| | | |
|---|---|---|
| **100.8** | **2.1** | Step over intermittent streambed on south slope of Rock Quarry Mountain |
| **101.2** | **1.7** | Step over small perennial stream. Campsite in hollow below |
| **101.7** | **1.2** | Enter thicker forest amid old pits dug for iron ore mining |
| **102.2** | **0.7** | Rock-hop Lanie Hollow Branch where valley has constricted |
| **102.9** | **0.0** | Reach US 278 and most northerly trailside parking. The PT is slated to continue north to meet Benton MacKaye Trail in Georgia |

## Pinhoti Trail Information

Alabama Trails Association
P.O. Box 371162
Birmingham, Alabama 35237
www.alabamatrailsasso.org

Talladega National Forest
www.r8web.com/alabama

Talladega National Forest
Shoal Creek Ranger District
450 Highway 46
Heflin, Alabama 36264
(256) 463-2272

Talladega Ranger District
1001 North Street
Highway 21 North
Talladega, Alabama 35150
(256) 362-2909

# WILD AZALEA TRAIL

At 26 miles, the Wild Azalea Trail is Louisiana's longest footpath. What it lacks in length, it makes up in beauty and biodiversity. Located in the Kisatchie National Forest, the trail runs from southeast to northwest. The trail was built in the early 1970s by Forest Service personnel and volunteer groups. No less than five ecosystems thrive here among the rolling pine-covered hills and lush bottomlands where clear waters flow over sandy streambeds beneath rich hardwoods. Also in these bottoms are wetlands, or bogs, locally known as bayous, where the elegant cypress tree reigns. Hickory and oak forests thrive in transitional zones, along with some of the largest dogwoods in the land. Don't let the Bayou State's reputation for flatness cloud your mind; the Wild Azalea Trail features plenty of vertical variation. Your legs will attest to this fact at the end of the day. Another surprise will be the wild character of the trail. The forest cover exudes a real sense of being "out there." And you really are. Only the beginning and end are developed.

The trail begins at the Woodworth Municipal Building, which offers safe parking, and follows along a quiet residential area before entering rich woods. From there, the path stays in heavily wooded-country, occasionally crossing forest roads. It continues through the bottomland along Clear Creek before climbing the first of many piney hills. Begin a series of surprisingly frequent ups and downs, culminating with the plunge into Castor Creek Scenic Area, where big trees form a cathedral hovering over the shady flats along the translucent waterway. A few more ascents and descents take you to LA 488 highway. The trail then winds beneath towering pines where the tap, tap, tap of the red-cockaded woodpecker is never far away. The often sparse understory of these pinelands contrasts greatly with the thick bottomlands. Pass the primitive Evangeline Camp, accessible only by foot, before dropping into another scenic area, the Wild Azalea Seep. This north-facing valley is on the Louisiana Natural Area Registry, and is home to several

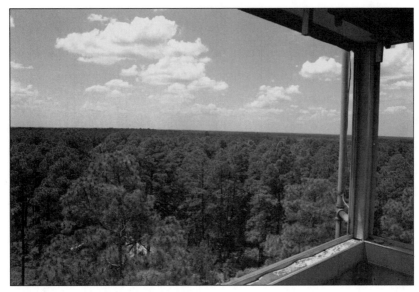

View from fire tower near Valentine Lake

species of orchids and other plants. Return to drier terrain before dipping into the Valentine Creek Valley, rife with wetlands. The trail makes one last special climb, up to the hill where Gardner Lookout Tower stands, offering a 360° view of the surrounding national forest and beyond. Just a mile further the Wild Azalea Trail ends at Valentine Lake Recreation Area.

Backpackers have many campsite options. The bottomlands of the streamsheds have flat tent sites, as well as water. Previously used campsites are located at 8.7, 12.7, 28.4, and 23.6 miles. Mosquitoes will be present at certain times of the year. They will be most numerous mid-spring through early summer, and following heavy rains during the warm season. But spring is a great time to visit, to see the trail's namesake azaleas in bloom, as well as the dogwoods and numerous wildflowers. Summer can be hot, but intrepid hikers can occasionally be spotted, trying to stay cool along the shady streambanks. Fall is highly recommended, as the mosquitoes have died down and the many deciduous trees put on a color show. Winter brings the most solitude. It isn't unusual to have mild, even spring-like weather in winter, and most of the larger streams are bridged, eliminating wet-footed crossings. This path will offer solitude any time of the year during the week, and on many weekends too. Be apprised that bicycles are allowed on the trail. Also, an Air Force training area is within earshot and sometimes jets can be heard and seen, streaking across the sky.

This yellow-blazed path is best hiked from southeast to northwest. The sun will mostly be at your back and the parking is very secure at Woodworth. The Wild Azalea Trail can be backpacked in its entirety in three days—a full weekend, if you start early on Friday. There is no need to resupply here. If the one-way distance is not long enough, consider making an out-and-back trek, doubling your distance and eliminating the necessity of bringing two cars or arranging a shuttle. There is no shuttle-for-pay operation here. The campground at Valentine Lake makes for a great turnaround spot, with its waterside campsites, potable water, showers, lake, and swimming area. Come to this swath of the Kisatchie National Forest with high expectations and you will not be disappointed, as the Wild Azalea Trail truly does show the wilder side of Louisiana.

# Wild Azalea Trail, Woodworth to Valentine Lake

| | |
|---|---|
| **Length:** | 26.3 miles |
| **Trail Condition:** | Excellent |
| **Highs:** | Castor Creek Scenic Area, Wild Azalea Seep, streamside bottomlands |
| **Lows:** | Mosquitoes |
| **Season:** | Year-round; best during early spring, fall, winter |
| **Difficulty:** | Moderate |
| **Use:** | Low to moderate |
| **Tips:** | Consider making a there-and-back hike for a full week trip. |
| **Campsites:** | 8.7, 12.7, 28.4, and 23.6 miles |

**WOODWORTH TRAILHEAD:** From the traffic circle in southwest Alexandria at the junction of US 165 and US 71, head south on US 165 for 9.3 miles to the small town of Woodworth and Castor Plunge Road (The left turn at this red light will be Robinson Bridge Road and the right turn will be Castor Plunge Road). Turn right at the red light and follow it 0.1 miles to the Woodworth Municipal Building, which will be on your left. Park here. The Wild Azalea Trail heads west on the concrete path leaving the parking area.

**VALENTINE LAKE TRAILHEAD:** From its junction with US 165 in Alexandria, head west on LA 28 for 13 miles to LA 121. Turn left on 121 and follow it for 0.3 miles, then turn left on Valentine Lake Road, FR 279. Follow FR 279 for 0.9 miles to reach FR 282. Turn right on FR 282 and follow it for 2.6 miles to reach the northwest Wild Azalea Trailhead.

The Wild Azalea Trail starts at the small, one-story Woodworth Municipal Building, which offers secure parking, as the police station is here. From the building, head west along a concrete sidewalk that runs alongside Castor Plunge Road. Soon, pass First Baptist Church and continue on through a quiet residential area where the friendly Louisianians are proud of their trail. At 0.7 miles, the path crosses Castor Plunge Road but continues its westerly course before petering out at Langston Road. Keep forward, now walking on the shoulder of Castor Plunge Road. Span Little Bayou on the road at mile 1.2, then leave the Woodworth city limits. Step over a cattle guard just after the pavement ends, then look right for the Wild Azalea Trail as it enters bona fide woodland at mile 1.7. You are now in the Kisatchie National Forest.

The trail immediately takes on a wild character as it traces the double yellow-painted blazes through the bottomland of Clear Creek. Tall pines stand guard over a forest of Southern magnolia, sweetgum, maple, and dogwood. Pass an upturned ancient jalopy beside the trail at mile 2.1. Skirt the edge of the valley, passing through an area with alternating sun and shade. Pine woods grow on the uphill side of the path. The trail veers left and briefly picks up an old logging grade before dipping down to cross a feeder branch of Clear Creek on a footbridge. The actual Clear Creek is bridged at mile 3.6 and is followed by a long boardwalk. A profusion of ferns thrives in these wet areas during the warm season. Also notice the smooth-trunked beech trees that prefer the cooler, moister conditions of these bottomlands. Leave the bottomland to climb and reach gravel FR 249 at mile 3.7.

Cross the forest road and descend, returning to more bottomland, then climb away to thinned-out pineland. Young longleaf pines and oaks are regenerating here among the scattered tall pines. Off in the distance, some pines with white bands are visible, evidence of red cockaded wood-pecker nesting sites. The nesting pine trees are also known as candle trees, as the sap pouring from the nest hole resembles wax dripping down a candle. The orange-banded trees in the area define the perimeters of the nest sites. Keep generally uphill to cross FR 208 at mile 4.8. You have now topped 200 feet in elevation. Veer slightly left along the road to re-enter thick woods. Pine woods like these need periodic fire to retain their natural state. Before man's intervention, lightning would often burn the understory of these pine stands. The bigger trees survive such burns. Now, forest personnel use prescribed burns to achieve the same result. Forest roads are often used as boundaries in delineating prescribed burns, so by simply crossing a forest road hikers will experience different forest conditions resulting from burns at different times. Look for black-ened bark along the lower sections of mature pine trees to indicate evi-dence of fire.

This section has a mix of pine and deciduous trees, such as red oak. The trail becomes fairly hilly as it passes over gated and little-used FR 2043. Swing around the dry upper drainage of Rocky Bayou. Pass through a clearing at mile 5.5. To your left is the water storage tank for the city of Alexandria. Descend among oaks before returning to piney hills and intersecting FR 212 at mile 6.1. Look left, walk just a short dis-tance, and re-enter recently burned woods. Dip down and rise to cross FR 287 at mile 7.1. Briefly pick up an old, grown-over roadbed, then descend into the valley of Loving Creek among oaks and hickories. The forest becomes more lush with sweetgum, maples, and azaleas as it nears Loving Creek. After a quick final drop, enter the bottomland and reach the clear stream at mile 7.5. This is a potential camping area. Notice the big magnolias, beech, and cypress trees, the latter with their knees protruding from the ground. Cane also thrives down here. Head downstream along Loving Creek, where seeps make the trailbed muddy. In places, the trailbed has been artificially raised with concrete block and gravel to assist in negotiating these wet areas.

Come alongside some bogs just before bridging Loving Creek at mile 8.2. Pick up an elevated roadbed that offers a good view of the junglesque bottomland to your right and a hillside to the left. Stay with the roadbed for half a mile, before abruptly veering left. Turn left with the blazes here—the old roadbed continues forward—but do not follow it. The next section of trail is the path's hilliest. Make a near U-turn around a hill and go up the watershed of Little Loving Creek, staying a good piece above an intermittent streambed. Cross the intermittent streambed at mile 8.4, climb over a small ridge, and cross little-used FR 2436, then descend to step over a tiny streamlet. Make a short, steep climb and quickly drop down to a mucky bottom and a bridge over another small creek at mile 8.7. Beyond this bridge is a good flat for camping.

Continuing on, climb away uphill, only to drop again to yet another bottom and a footbridge spanning Little Loving Creek at mile 8.9. Climb away from Little Loving Creek in more open woods. As you pass along the trail, small lizards will skitter noisily away among the dry leaves. Cross FR 241 at mile 9.3. Keep climbing beyond the road on a wide trailbed beneath a pine plantation. Veer right off the wide trail into a hardwood-dominated forest and descend to Long Branch, another clear, sand-bottomed stream, at mile 9.9. This is an exceptionally beautiful valley with huge beech trees. Briefly head upstream, then curve back around down the valley in drier terrain on the edge of the bottom, dropping back down to the water's edge at mile 10.5. Keep along the creek, where a huge flat lies to your right. This area is heavily punctuated with wetlands and bogs, some of which have been created by beavers. Expect to see beaver dams in the area that may flood the trailbed. Cypress trees become more prevalent.

Briefly head upstream, then climb away from the creek, staying with the yellow blazes into higher, drier terrain. Once atop the hill, make an abrupt left turn before arriving at FR 273 at mile 12.0. Cross the forest road, then work your way down toward Castor Creek. Many holly trees and a few cedar trees grace the trailside here. You are now entering the Castor Creek Scenic Area, a 90-acre parcel at the junction of Brushy and Castor creeks. Massive loblolly pines tower over gum, ash, oak, and beech trees. Span the wide, shallow stream at mile 12.7. Continue through bottomland beyond the bridge. Wet weather drainages bisect the trail from the hillside to the north. Turn away from the streamshed and undulate through open woods toward Cypress Creek. Drop steeply to a feeder stream of Cypress Branch and bridge the unnamed watercourse at mile 13.6. Ascend from the thickness into open pine-oak woods to emerge at a power line. Veer right under the line and re-enter the woods, soon dropping into a rich and attractive ravine. At the bottom lies Cypress Branch, which the trail bridges at mile 14.0. An elevated trailbed makes for easier going through the wettest spots.

Ascend back into pine-oak woods, carefully staying with the yellow blazes. Achieve a ridgeline and cruise through young pine woods. Dive off the ridge and circle around the upper drainage of Cypress Branch, winding in and out of a hardwood forest. Span a normally dry streambed on a footbridge before heading uphill among pure pine woods towering over grass and brush to reach paved FR 273 at mile 15.0. Cross the forest road and immediately come to a trailhead parking area. A few steps to the north is blacktopped LA 488. To continue the Wild Azalea Trail, cross blacktopped LA 488, but keep on the same side, the east side, of FR 273 at the trailhead parking area.

Look for the yellow blazes and enter pine woods with a brushy understory of young trees higher than a person's head. Many young longleaf pines grow here, with thin trunks sprouting skyward, usually not branching out until they are 5 or 6 feet tall. Very young longleafs look like pine bushes sprouting from the ground. Undulate through hilly country. At mile 15.8, pick up a closed jeep road and follow it about 50 yards before angling left beneath mature pine trees. The wide path shows less use than the section south of LA 488. At mile 16.1, dip off the pine ridge into the upper valley of Boggy Bayou. This area is not boggy, rather it is a shallow valley-head thick with oaks and hickories and no running stream in it. Steep hillsides flank the valley. Pass an odd relic of wood posts emerging from the ground and head out of the valley as the trail nearly doubles back on itself to reach the piney ridgeline. Watch for the white-banded pine trees.

At mile 17.1, reach FR 273. Turn left and follow the road southward a bit to reach a gravel trailhead parking area on your right. Pass through the fenceline. Just ahead is a vault toilet. The trail continuing forward heads to Evangeline Camp. The official portion of the Wild Azalea Trail veers right, just before the vault toilet, and soon comes to a concrete pad, part of the old camp bathroom. To your left is a defunct pump well and beyond it is Evangeline Camp, beneath an oak copse looking over a grassy meadow. This is a good camp but has no nearby water since the pump well was dismantled.

The Wild Azalea Trail continues downhill from the concrete pad into a shallow valley on a wide, sandy path. Pass a grove of young longleaf pines before entering a thicker forest of hardwoods and some pines. You are now entering the Wild Azalea Seep, listed on the Louisiana Natural Area Registry. The path stays on the margin of the dense seep vegetation. A small bridge passes over the watercourse. Magnolias grow tall here. There are many orchids in the 123-acre area and the only known population of bog moss west of the Mississippi River. Climb away steeply on a raised trailbed, working to surmount the ridge between the Wild Azalea Seep and Lamotte Creek. The trail is now heading westward. Water bars have been placed on the trail here to minimize erosion. Come to Lamotte Creek at mile 18.4, as it makes a sharp curve beside a steep hill. Good campsites are in the flat here. Bridge the stream, climb along a narrow ridgeline, and soon reach a trail junction. The blue-blazed Lamotte Spur Trail leads right for 2.6 miles to the Lakeshore Trail on Kincaid Lake.

Continue forward on the Wild Azalea Trail, mostly ascending through an open forest heavy with dogwoods. Dip into a shallow valley head on a sandy path just before crossing Fr 240 at mile 18.9. Cross the road and come to a second trail junction at mile 19.1. The Kincaid Spur Trail, also known as the Wild Azalea Spur Trail, leads right for 2 miles to the Kincaid Recreation Area entry station. Keep southwest on the Wild Azalea Trail, skirting the valley of Mack Branch amidst oak woods. Cross a couple of gated and growing-over forest roads, keeping parallel with Mack Branch, and start a pattern of dipping into shallow coves and moderately ascending over pine ridges. Pass some intermittent stream-beds before bridging the headwater streambed of Mack Branch at mile 20.7. This section of Mack Branch is often dry. Turn away from Mack Branch and trace an old road alongside a rusty barbed wire fence ascending a pine ridge. Pass a cluster of woodpecker nests just before coming to paved FR 279 at mile 21.1. Cross the road and keep westerly through pine-oak woods. This woodland gives way to mature pine trees with a thick understory of maple and sweetgum. The forest changes again as the trail dips into the Valentine Creek valley. Climb away from this dry streambed then dip into a thick narrow bottomland along a perennial feeder stream that is traversed on a raised trailbed at mile 22.1.

Leave this lush valley, where ferns grow waist high, and once again parallel a fence line, dipping into another intermittent feeder branch. Head up this valley to cross a logging road, then pick up long abandoned roadbed that descends into Long Creek, an attractive watercourse that feeds Valentine Creek. There is a good campsite here under a beech tree, on the inside of a bend in the translucent stream. Head upstream beyond the campsite and span Long Branch at mile 23.7. Sharply climb a hill then veer right on an old road. Skirt the hillside before dipping into the Valentine Creek Valley, which is resplendent with bogs in its bottomland. Pass through these swamps on a raised trailbed before bridging another wetland. Come to Valentine Creek at mile 24.6 and cross this wide watercourse on a sturdy bridge. Work away from the bottomland on an old roadbed, ascending a dry cove, leaving the valley and entering pure

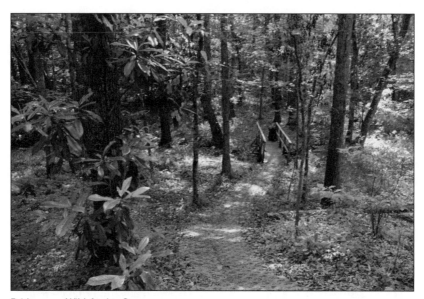

Bridge over Wild Azalea Seep

pine woods. Work your way uphill, topping out at a clearing and the Gardner Lookout Tower at mile 25.9. Climb the tower and enjoy a 360-degree view of the surrounding forestland and distant water towers of the adjacent communities.

Descend the tower and cross FR 288. Follow the yellow blazes along a jeep road. Pass under a telephone line and veer left away from the road as the path narrows. Come alongside FR 282. At mile 26.3, come to a trail junction. Ahead, the white-blazed Valentine Lake Nature Trail leads 0.9 miles around the south shore of Valentine Lake and to the north loop of the campground. The Wild Azalea Trail turns right and ends in the parking area just a few feet away. This parking area may be closed in winter, necessitating the use of the nature trail to access the year-round parking area in the north.

## Wild Azalea Trail Log

### WOODWORTH TO VALENTINE LAKE

| | | |
|---|---|---|
| 0.0 | 26.3 | Beginning of Wild Azalea Trail at Woodworth Town Hall |
| 0.7 | 25.6 | Cross Castor Plunge Road |
| 1.2 | 25.1 | Span Little Bayou on Castor Plunge Road |
| 1.7 | 24.6 | Leave road and enter woods of Kisatchie National Forest. |
| 3.6 | 22.7 | Bridge Clear Creek on footbridge followed by long boardwalk |
| 3.7 | 22.6 | Reach gravel FR 249, keep in hills |
| 4.8 | 21.5 | Cross FR 208 |
| 6.1 | 20.2 | Cross FR 212, trail rolls up and down |
| 7.1 | 19.2 | Cross FR 287 and descend into the valley of Loving Creek |
| 8.2 | 18.1 | Bridge Loving Creek and stay in valley on old roadbed, then turn up Little Loving Creek Valley, heading up and down small feeder-stream valleys |
| 8.9 | 17.4 | Span Little Loving Creek |
| 9.3 | 17.0 | Cross FR 241 into pines then descend to Long Branch valley with many wetlands |
| 12.0 | 14.3 | Leave valley and climb to reach FR 273. Descend toward Castor Creek |
| 12.7 | 13.6 | Bridge Castor Creek in attractive bottomland and head toward Cypress Branch |
| 14.0 | 12.3 | Bridge Cypress Branch, an elevated trailbed traverses wettest spots in valley |

## Wild Azalea Trail Log *(continued)*

| | | |
|---|---|---|
| **15.0** | **11.3** | Reach FR 273. Cross forest road and reach trailhead parking area beside LA 488. Cross LA 488 and enter tall pine forest |
| **16.0** | **10.3** | Dip off the pine ridge into the upper valley of Boggy Bayou. Quickly leave valley as the trail nearly doubles back and returns to pine ridge |
| **17.1** | **9.2** | Reach FR 273. Turn left and follow road to reach a gravel trailhead parking area on your right. Pass through the fenceline across FR 273, and soon reach Evangeline Camp. Descend toward Wild Azalea Seep |
| **18.4** | **7.9** | Reach Lamotte Creek, bridge stream, climb a bit to reach trail junction. Blue-blazed Lamotte Spur Trail leads right for 2.6 miles to Kincaid Lake |
| **18.9** | **7.4** | Crossing FR 240 |
| **19.1** | **7.2** | Trail junction, Kincaid Spur Trail leads right 2 miles to Kincaid Recreation Area entry station. Wild Azalea Trail skirts valley of Mack Branch |
| **20.7** | **5.6** | Bridge the headwater streambed of Mack Branch |
| **21.1** | **5.2** | Cross paved FR 279. Keep westerly through pine-oak woods |
| **23.7** | **2.6** | Cross Long Branch in attractive bottomland |
| **24.6** | **1.7** | Reach Valentine Creek, many bogs around. Cross creek on wide footbridge, climb into pine woods |
| **25.9** | **0.4** | Gardner Lookout Tower, 360° views. Shortly cross FR 288 |
| **26.3** | **0.0** | Trail junction, white-blazed Valentine Lake Nature Trail leads 0.9 miles around the south shore of Valentine Lake and to the north loop of Valentine Lake Campground. Wild Azalea Trail turns right and ends in the parking area just a few feet away. |

## Wild Azalea Trail Information

Kisatchie National Forest Supervisor's Office
2500 Shreveport Highway
Pineville, Louisiana 71360-2009
(318) 473-7160
www.southernregion.fs.fed.us/kisatchie

Calcasieu Ranger District
9912 Highway 28 West
Boyce, Louisiana 71360
(318) 793-9427

# LONG TRAILS CHECKLIST

**C**heck off every trail segment you have hiked in this book. When you have hiked them all, visit www.johnnymolloy.com and e-mail Johnny. He will then issue you a certificate of achievement for being a bona fide long trail hiker!

## BARTRAM TRAIL

__ Russell Bridge to Warwoman Dell

__ Warwoman Dell to
Hale Ridge Road

__ Hale Ridge Road to
Buckeye Creek

__ Buckeye Creek to Wallace Branch

__ Wallace Branch to
Nantahala Lake

__ Nantahala Lake to Winding Stairs

__ Winding Stairs to Cheoah Bald

## BENTON MACKAYE TRAIL

__ Springer Mtn. to
Little Skeenah Creek

__ Little Skeenah Creek to
Shallowford Bridge

__ Shallowford Bridge to
Bushy Head Gap

__ Bushy Head Gap to Watson Gap

__ Watson Gap to Ocoee River

## BLACK CREEK TRAIL

__ Fairley Bridge Ldg. to Janice Ldg.

__ Janice Ldg. to Big Creek Ldg

## FLORIDA TRAIL

*Big Cypress National Preserve*

__ Loop Road to Tamiami Trail

__ Tamiami Trail to I-75

*Ocala National Forest*

__ Clearwater Lake to
Juniper Springs

__ Juniper Springs to Salt Springs Is.

__ Salt Springs Island to
Rodman Dam

*Apalachicola National Forest*

__ Medart to Bradwell Bay

__ Bradwell Bay to Porter Lake

__ Porter Lake to Vilas

__ Vilas to Estiffanulga

## FOOTHILLS TRAIL

__ Oconee State Park to
Burrells Ford

__ Burrells Ford to Bad Creek Access

__ Bad Creek Access to
Rocky Bottom

__ Rocky Bottom to Jones Gap S. P.

## PINHOTI TRAIL

__ Porters Gap to Cheaha State Park

__ Cheaha State Park to Cleburne

__ Cleburne to Coleman Lake

__ Coleman Lake to East Dugger Mt.

__ East Dugger Mt. to High Point

## WILD AZALEA TRAIL

__ Woodworth to Valentine Lake

# INDEX

# ABOUT THE AUTHOR

Johnny Molloy is an outdoor writer based in Tennessee. He was born in Memphis and moved to Knoxville in 1980 to attend the University of Tennessee. In Knoxville he developed his love of the natural world that has since become the primary focus of his life.

His career started on a backpacking foray into the Great Smoky Mountains National Park. That first trip, though a disaster, unleashed an innate love of the outdoors that has led to Molloy averaging over 100 nights in the wild per year since 1982, backpacking and canoe camping throughout the United States and abroad. In the lofty mountains of the Smokies alone, he has spent over 650 nights cultivating his woodsmanship and outdoor's expertise.

In 1987, after graduating from the University of Tennessee with a degree in economics, he continued to spend an ever-increasing time in natural places, becoming more skilled in a variety of outdoor environments. Friends enjoyed his adventure stories, one even suggested he write a book. Soon, he was parlaying his love of the outdoors into an occupation. The results of his efforts are books covering his home state of Tennessee and much of the United States: *Day & Overnight Hikes in the Great Smoky Mountains National Park* (Menasha Ridge Press, 1995 & 2001); *Trial by Trail: Backpacking in the Smoky Mountains* (University of Tennessee Press, 1996); *The Best in Tent Camping: Southern Appalachians and Smoky Mountains* (Menasha Ridge Press, 1997, 1999, & 2001); *Best in Tent Camping: Florida* (Menasha Ridge Press, 1998 & 2001); *Day & Overnight Hikes in Shenandoah National Park* (Menasha Ridge Press, 1998); *Beach & Coastal Camping in Florida* (University Press of Florida, 1999); *The Best in Tent Camping: Colorado* (Menasha Ridge Press, 1999 & 2001); *A Paddler's Guide to Everglades National Park* (University Press of Florida, 2000); *Day & Overnight Hikes in the Monongahela National Forest* (Menasha Ridge Press, 2000); *The Best in Tent Camping: West Virginia* (Menasha Ridge Press, 2000); *Mount*

*Rogers Outdoor Recreation Area Handbook* (Menasha Ridge Press, 2001); *Hiking Trails of Florida's National Forests, Parks, and Preserves* (University Press of Florida, 2001); *60 Hikes within 60 Miles: Nashville* (Menasha Ridge Press, 2002); *From the Swamp to the Keys: A Paddle Through Florida History* (University Press of Florida, 2002); *Land Between the Lakes Outdoor Recreation Handbook* (Menasha Ridge Press, 2003). Molloy has also written numerous articles for magazines such as *Backpacker* and *Sea Kayaker.* He also has written for web sites such as Gorp.com. He continues to write and travel extensively to all four corners of the United States, finding adventure in a variety of outdoor pursuits.